SEX CONFESSIONS OF A YOUNG BLONDE SCUBA DIVING INSTRUCTOR ON A DIVE TRIP (24 YEARS OLD)

SEX CONFESSIONS OF A YOUNG BLONDE SCUBA DIVING INSTRUCTOR ON A DIVE TRIP (24 YEARS OLD)

I Didn't Dive Because 14 Old Men Forced Me to Be the Submissive Sex Pet & Gear Slave of the Whole Dive Resort

My Sex Confessions - The Series

DELISHA KEANE

www.DelishaKeane.com

Sex Confessions of a Young Blonde Scuba Diving Instructor on a Dive Trip (24 Years Old): I Didn't Dive Because 14 Old Men Forced Me to Be the Submissive Sex Pet & Gear Slave of the Whole Dive Resort

2nd edition

My Sex Confessions - The Series

ISBN (print) 979-8-87-280246-4

v1.0

To Mom & Dad:
Thank you for supporting my appetite for sexual experimentation - from my teenage years to today!

To YOU!
Thank you for supporting me as a writer and for motivating me in my sexual experiments.

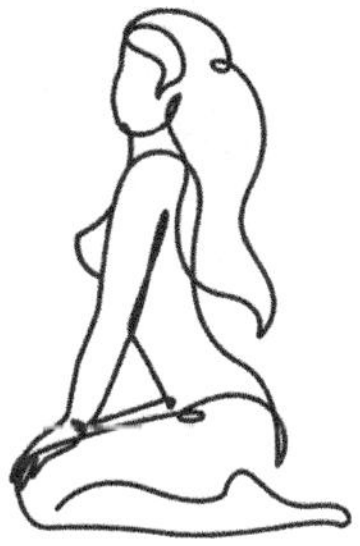

Contents - Sex Confessions

PHASE I
Before The Trip

1

Preparing For My Dive Trip as a Fuck Doll on a Sperm-Only Diet

Finally! Today, Saturday, is the start of a week-long sex & scuba vacation with 14 old men. I will be on a sperm-only diet, dependent on the men to feed me with their semen delivery hoses. And my young mid-20 blonde female body will be nothing more than a sex object, a plaything for them to satisfy their most primal, bestial male sexual urges that marriage sex cannot provide to them.

Conversations in the sex confessions published in this diary have been abridged to make it flow easier for you, and well... Because my memory is not perfect, especially when I am aroused!

THIS MORNING, I stood in the beach condo where I live, admiring the ocean view that stretched out beyond the floor-to-ceiling windows. The place isn't mine, and I am grateful to the old man who let me use it for free just because he loves fucking me when he visits. I felt a thrill at the thought of that old man, a friend of my Daddy, who masturbated to images of me since my teenage years.

As I prepared for the dive trip with 14 other older men, my mind raced with anticipation. These cock-carrying beasts will be using me to satisfy their darkest sexual desires, and I couldn't wait. In my head, I could see their eager faces as they looked upon my naked body, ready to take what they wanted from me. The thought sent shivers down my spine, and I felt my pussy tingle with excitement.

"God, I can't wait to be their fuck toy," I whispered to myself, biting my lip as I imagined the rough hands of those men gripping my body, sliding over my exposed flesh and exploring every inch of me as if I were a mere object for them to play with.

I moved around the condo, gathering my things for the trip. My heart pounded in my chest, my breathing quickened, and I could feel my nipples harden beneath my skimpy tank top.

"Fourteen men, all wanting to use me... I must be the luckiest girl in the world," I thought, smiling wickedly to myself as I imagined each one of them taking turns with me, pounding into my wet, willing cunt, their grunts and moans filling the air as they reached their climax.

"Maybe they'll even fight over me," I mused, delighting in the thought of being the center of a primal struggle between these men, each one desperate to claim me for their own.

I just hoped these men wouldn't be shy about using me. Many men are. I often have to repeat a few times before men understand what I mean by letting them use me in any way they want.

As I continued to prepare for the trip, I had a hard time keeping my focus on preparing to meet them at the Miami airport to begin our week of debauchery together.

"Let's make sure they know what they're getting," I said to myself as I picked up a bottle of nail polish. I carefully painted the letters SPERMIVORE on my toenails, making sure each letter faced away from me so that anyone looking at them would be able to read it perfectly.

"Perfect," I thought, admiring my handiwork. "Now everyone will know that I'm a special kind of creature eating nothing but men's semen."

My mind raced with thoughts of being on my knees, lips wrapped around thick, throbbing cocks, sucking hungrily, and greedily swallowing every drop of cum offered to me.

"God, just thinking about spending an entire week as a submissive cum slut is making me wet," I admitted to myself, feeling a shiver of anticipation raced down my spine.

After painting my toenails, I rummaged through my recent purchases to find the perfect footwear for this trip: high-platform sandals I had ordered specifically for this sexual dive adventure. They were far from comfortable, but I knew they'd make my ass wiggle just right, driving those men wild.

"Who needs comfort when you're a walking sex object?" I mused while slipping them on my feet, admiring the colorful anklets that adorned the top of the sandals. I felt a sense of pride in knowing that my purpose was to please and arouse old men.

For years now, old men's cocks have become my gods, and my purpose in life was to worship them.

My gaze shifted to the mirror as I assessed my outfit, wondering if it would be enough to satiate the desires of the 14 men I'd be joining at the airport. First, I looked at the drawstring shorts hugging my hips, the thin material barely covering my pussy. The narrow waistband exposed the curve of my lower abdomen, almost like an arrow pointing to the pussy that would be theirs all week. One side of the shorts opened widely, revealing I wore no panties, just as I never did.

I ran my fingers along the strings holding the shorts together, contemplating how much I could tease them by wearing such provocative attire. The thought of being their object of desire fueled my excitement.

"Fourteen hungry pairs of eyes devouring every inch of me," I whispered, feeling my arousal grow at the prospect of parading myself in front of them like a walking feast.

As I stood there in my platform sandals and barely-there shorts, I could almost hear their approving whispers and feel their lustful gazes. I couldn't wait to give myself over to their desires completely, to be their willing, submissive plaything.

As I continued to admire myself in the mirror, my gaze shifted to the lace-up tank top I wore. The tiny garment barely covered the bottom part of my boobs, leaving my flat belly fully exposed. The openings around the arms were wide, and the entire front was a drawstring that matched the one on my shorts, creating a sinfully tantalizing ensemble.

"Perfect," I thought, feeling more like a sex object than ever before. "This should make old cocks vibrate with desire."

The pieces of fabric over my tits ended just past my nipples, held together by a drawstring. I imagined the men's eyes feasting on the sight before them, my body an irresistible invitation for their bestial urges.

"Will they be pleased with their living, breathing fuck doll?"

I reveled in the thought of being the center of their attention, their lusty gazes and rough touches driving me wild with desire. For a week. A whole week! Every fiber of my being wanted to honor these old men, to fulfill my role as the ultimate cock-pleasuring device—a thing they casually use to masturbate.

"Time to pack," I thought, my gaze lingering on the backpack lying empty on the floor. It was astonishing how little I needed for this trip, considering my main purpose was to be a sex object on a hot tropical island. Grinning, I began filling the bag with the few items that would help me fulfill their desires.

First, I packed the clothes I purchased after getting feedback from pervs (I mean, fans!) supporting me on my sexual exploration journey.

Then I filled the backpack with whatever bondage gear would fit in, including handcuffs, nipple clamps, ankle restraints, a chocker, a leash, a butt plug, and the 5-inch dildo ball gag I discovered during clit torturing sessions. I wanted to give the men free rein over my body, letting them bind me and use me however they pleased. The possibilities were endless, and I couldn't wait to find out how much they would dare to do with the young naked chick in their claws.

Finally, I added a bottle of lube, knowing that my butthole would be a prized item on their menu. The thought of a series of thick, Viagra-hardened cocks stretching my tight hole sent my body quivering, and I clenched my teeth in anticipation, especially since I was sure that a few of these married men had never fucked a woman up the ass, although they fantasized about it for most of their life. It seems to be the case with all old married men.

"Will they be rough enough?" I pondered, biting my lip. Often, men talk a good game, but they need encouragement or reassurance to really let loose and go wild on me. My mind drifted as I envisioned a series of violent sexual acts they could perform if they truly decided to use me as a fuck doll.

They could grab me with rough hands and pin me down as they took turns thrusting their hard cocks into every hole of mine. I could almost already feel their thick rods stretching me, making me scream in pleasure and pain. My wrists could be bound above my head so that I couldn't escape, my body owned by a pack of wolves ravaging my young, naked, and vulnerable body without mercy.

They could line up one after the other until they've filled every inch of me with cum, leaving me a writhing mess of blissful agony—used and discarded like a ragdoll. All throughout this agonizingly sweet torture, I'd be enticed by their raw animalistic power. Call me whatever you want, I crave being a willing sex object—a plaything old men use and abuse as they desire.

My arousal intensified with each depraved fantasy, my wetness dripping between my legs in anticipation of what was to come.

"Enough daydreaming," I told myself, shaking off my lustful thoughts. "Time to head to the airport."

I decided to leave my SUV at the condo and called for an Uber ride, my pulse racing with anticipation as I waited for its arrival.

"Fourteen old men," I murmured one last time before getting into the car. "I can't wait to be at their mercy for a full week."

I'VE OBSERVED *that men have a variety of preferences for different aspects of my sexual experiences, so I am organizing and publishing my journal entries according to common themes for easier selection, access, and enjoyment.*

My published sex life diaries range from mild exhibitionism to violent gang bangs. If you visit my author website at delishakeane.com, you can browse through the various sexual confessions and find the ones that are more likely to get your cock hard - oops! I mean, suit your particular preferences. Naked hugs & wet kisses!

2

Teasing The Old Cock of My Uber Driver as Practice

My heart fluttered with excitement as I settled into the backseat of the Uber, my backpack resting on my lap. My eyes roamed over the driver's reflection in the rearview mirror. He was an older man, exactly the type carrying my god between his legs. I couldn't help but smile, taking it as a good omen for the filthy, sex-filled week ahead of me.

"Nice day, isn't it?" I said casually, breaking the silence that had filled the car since my entrance.

"Indeed," he replied, his eyes meeting mine in the mirror for a brief moment before focusing back on the road. "Where are you headed?"

"An island for a week-long scuba diving trip," I replied, smirking. "But it's not just any trip... It'll be with 14 older gentlemen as their personal fuck doll."

His eyes widened, clearly taken aback by my brazen admission. I could sense his curiosity piqued as he struggled to maintain focus on the road.

"Yep," I continued, speaking slowly and deliberately. "I'll be their plaything for the whole week, letting them use my body however they desire. They can take turns fucking me, or even all at once if they want. My young little cunt, my hungry mouth, and my tight ass will be theirs to abuse as they please."

A silence settled over the car as the driver tried to process what I had just revealed. I could tell he was shocked, but then again, that was exactly my intention. I was already having fun and hadn't even reached the airport to start the vacation!

"Every day and night, they can make me swallow their massive cocks, fuck me so hard I can barely walk, and cover me in their hot, sticky cum," I said, relishing every crude word that spilled from my lips. "And the best part? I'll only eat sperm for the entire week—no food, just their delicious loads filling my belly."

"Are... are you serious? An escort?" the driver stammered, stealing a glance at me as if trying to determine if I was joking.

"No! Not getting paid a penny," I clarified, a wicked smile spreading across my face. "I can't think of anything more satisfying than being a willing cum dumpster for old men. Worshipping old cocks and swallowing their seed is like a religion to me."

The tension in the car was palpable as the driver grappled with my explicit confession. His knuckles whitened on the steering wheel, and I couldn't help but notice the growing bulge in his pants. The thought of how I'd just affected him sent a shiver down my spine as my own arousal intensified.

"Wow," he muttered, still seemingly at a loss for words. "That's... that's quite the trip."

I raised an eyebrow, sensing his disbelief. "You think I'm joking?" I asked, my voice low and sultry. "Trust me, there's nothing I enjoy more than to be used by depraved old men in any way they see fit."

"Really?" he asked, one hand gripping the steering wheel tight as if trying to regain control of the situation.

I nodded eagerly, relishing in his discomfort. "I don't like a gentle touch," I purred, "I want them to tie me up and take turns using my body like a piece of meat. Force me to be their little slut; use my body like it's theirs for the taking. Force their cocks down my throat until

I'm begging for air and leave my ass blazing hot from spanking. Pound into me relentlessly until I can't walk straight for days. And when they're finally done, I'll eagerly swallow every last drop of their cum, not wasting a single bit. A girl needs protein, after all."

"Wow, you really are something else," he said, his voice thick with desire. I noticed the bulge in his pants growing larger, straining against the fabric. The sight filled me with a sense of power and excitement.

"Thank you," I replied coyly, reveling in his obvious arousal. "You know, I sometimes wonder if there's a single man out there who could resist fucking me if I offered myself to him. But so far, I haven't found one yet."

"Here's our exit," the driver eventually said, driving off the highway at the airport entrance, his bulge still prominent, a testament to the power of my words and the raw, unbridled sexuality I exuded.

"You don't believe me, do you? God, I wish I could just strip down for you right now," I sighed, my voice dripping with desire. "Just to show you how much of a sex object I could be for you also." I bit my lip seductively, looking him up and down as he tried to keep his eyes on the road.

He glanced over at me, clearly struggling to maintain his composure. "You're really something else, aren't you?"

"Unfortunately, it's not that easy," I confessed, twirling a strand of my blonde hair around my finger, remembering the first time I got naked in an Uber. "These shorts and tank top have drawstrings that take forever to adjust in front of a mirror. Otherwise, I'd be more than happy to get naked for you."

His knuckles tightened on the steering wheel, betraying his lustful thoughts. "So if I asked you to strip, you're saying you would?"

"Absolutely," I purred, devouring him with my eyes. "But as I said, these damn drawstrings make it impossible to do so quickly."

I could see his mind racing, picturing all the dirty things he could do to me if given the chance. His fingers drummed on the wheel, contemplating the possibilities.

"Maybe next time I'll wear something a little more... practical," I suggested wickedly, imagining myself in a short skimpy sundress with nothing underneath and deep cleavage.

"Next time, huh?" he managed to choke out, his voice thick with desire.

"Definitely," I confirmed, feeling a shiver of excitement run down my spine.

"Alright," the Uber driver finally said, a challenging glint in his eyes. "If you're not just bullshitting me, then how about this? On your return trip, call me for a ride back."

I couldn't help but grin at his boldness, feeling a spark of excitement ignite within me. So he thought I was bluffing, did he?

"Deal," I agreed, completely confident in my ability to follow through on my promise. "You'll be surprised when I call, I assure you."

He raised an eyebrow, skepticism still evident on his face. "We'll see," he replied, seemingly unconvinced.

"Here," I said, pulling out my phone and handing it to him once we stopped at the terminal. "Put in your cell number, and I'll make sure to call you directly for my ride back."

He hesitated for a moment before taking my phone, inputting his number, and returning it to me. I could sense his anticipation mixed with doubt as he tried to gauge whether or not I was serious about our little arrangement.

My mind raced with thoughts of how I would fulfill my end of the bargain. I imagined myself in a flimsy sundress, my bare breasts and waxed pussy hidden beneath the thin material. The idea of stripping down in front of a stranger, exposing every inch of my body to his hungry gaze, had me practically throbbing with desire. I knew this man would be no different from the others I'd encountered—once he saw what I had to offer, he'd be unable to resist using me for his own pleasure, and I could add his cock to the list of gods I'd worshipped.

"Remember," I warned him playfully, "don't be too shocked when you get that call."

"Guess I'll have to see it to believe it," he shot back, smirking.

With that, I turned and sauntered into the airport, leaving him sitting in his car with wide eyes, stunned. I knew our next encounter would be a lot of fun.

3

Meeting The 14 Old Men at The Gate & Establishing Brutal Sex Rules

I strutted through the Miami airport, my provocative outfit drawing gazes from men and women alike. My nipples were clearly visible through the tight top, and my ass cheeks peeked out from beneath the ridiculously short shorts. I relished in the attention, enjoying the fact that each pair of eyes on me fed my insatiable hunger for sex and desire.

As I approached our departure gate, anticipation bubbled inside me. This scuba & sex trip would be a week-long feast for my lustful appetite, and I could hardly wait to meet the 14 older men who'd flown down from up North just to indulge their carnal cravings with me. They'd been on a layover, transferring flights at the Miami airport. I was joining them for the final leg of our journey.

When I finally spotted the group, I felt a familiar tingle between my legs—that delicious ache for pleasure and submission. I watched as Ralph, the divemaster and trip leader, recognized me and alerted the others. Their eyes devoured me like ravenous wolves stalking prey, and I reveled in it.

"Boys," Ralph called out as I approached, "our fuck doll has arrived." The men's eyes locked onto me like hungry vultures, and a shiver of pleasure coursed through my veins. This was exactly what I craved—to be their prey, their willing fuck toy. And I was thrilled to see that Ralph had fully understood what I wanted, as I had explained to him when organizing the trip.

"Hi there, boys," I purred, making my way around the group, hugging each man tightly, pressing my breasts against their chests, and lifting one leg suggestively every once in a while. As I moved from embrace to embrace, I caught snippets of hushed conversation among the men.

"Damn, she's even hotter in person..."

"Can't believe we're gonna have a whole week with her..."

"Damn, she's a perfect 10..."

"God, look at that ass..."

"Is this real? Fuck, we're in for a wild week..."

Their crude remarks only fueled my desire for the debauchery that awaited us. After all, I have always loved being seen as a sex object from as far as I could remember, even in my teenage years, and this trip had been organized specifically for me to indulge in my wildest fantasies.

The owner of the dive shop where I used to work in my hometown had been very open to the idea. Of course, the numerous blowjobs I gave in when I worked for him probably helped!

My heart raced as three familiar faces stepped forward during the introductions. Theo, Harvey, and Fred—I hadn't recognized them on the video call we held to plan the trip, but now, I remembered them from a dive trip a few years ago when I was just an innocent 18-year-old dive instructor. It seemed like an eternity ago, although it had only been six years. My eyes widened as memories flooded my mind.

"Delisha, you remember us, don't you?" Theo growled, the hunger in his voice unmistakable. "We were on that trip where we forced you down, tore off your clothes, and examined your sexy young body and juicy pussy like it was our own personal toy."

“Such a shame none of us got to fuck you back then,” Fred added, smirking. “But that’s why we’re here now, isn’t it?”

“Every night since that trip, I’ve dreamed of fucking you,” Theo confessed, licking his lips. “Almost every night, you know... And now, I finally get my chance!”

Their words gave me shivers, knowing I had awakened their primal sexual instincts a few years ago and that they still craved me to this day. The memories of being forcefully stripped and held down by these men made my pussy pulse with anticipation.

“Alright, gentlemen,” I said, commanding their attention once more. “Now that we’re all acquainted, let’s review the rules for the week. We went over some of them on our video call, but I’ve added a few more to ensure we all have an unimaginable time.” They leaned in, eager to hear what new depravities awaited them.

Some of you, pervs (oops! I mean, fans!), told me the list of rules was a bit long. Well, as I mentioned before, I often have to “spell it out,” over and over, that you can abuse my body. Unless I state it, repeat it, and insist, most men quickly revert back to being gentlemen. So, I had prepared these “rules” as a way to “spell it out.”

And some of the rules were just for fun, of course!

“FIRST, thank you all for completing your health checks as discussed on the call,” I began, appreciating their commitment to safety. The men nodded in agreement, their eyes never leaving my body.

“Alright, boys,” I continued, my voice sultry and dripping with promise. “Let’s talk about the first rule.”

There was silence in the group as they hung on my every word.

“During this week,” I explained, “I will only eat sperm and water. That means each of you must feed me three times a day—yes, with your cocks in my mouth. We’re looking at about one liter of semen in total.”

Their eyes widened, and several jaws dropped as they processed my words. One man chuckled nervously, while another managed to say, "Damn, girl, that's... a lot of sucking!"

"Isn't it?" I replied with a sly smile, relishing their reactions. "But that's what I want—to be used, fucked, and filled with all your delicious seed."

Spending a full week on a semen-only diet was the main reason for me to have organized that trip with my former employer.

I could feel my own arousal building at the thought, and it seemed the men were sharing in my excitement. Whispers erupted among them, crude comments about how they would gladly fill me up with their hot, sticky loads.

"Second rule," I continued, raising a finger for emphasis. "All week, I will wear a butt plug." The men exchanged intrigued glances, some grinning in anticipation. "You can do anything you want to me, but my tight little asshole is reserved for the last night. It'll be a special treat for all of us."

"Can't wait to pop your ass, fuck doll," one man said, his voice husky with desire.

"Better get that plug extra large then," another chimed in, making everyone chuckle.

As the laughter subsided, I could see the fire in their eyes growing wilder, and I started to believe this group of men could be a group capable of unleashing their darkest desires upon me. And I couldn't have been more eager to let them.

"Alright, guys," I said, my voice dripping with anticipation. "Time for the third rule." The men leaned in closer, eager to hear more. "You all have your cabins—two per cabin, right? Well, I don't get one. Instead, I'll spend one night in each of your cabins, giving you and your roommate a full night to do anything you want with me." Their eyes widened, and I smirked at their reactions. "Except for anal, of course. That's reserved for our last night together."

"Fuck yeah," one man growled, his erection straining against his pants. "Can't wait to use that sweet body of yours all night long."

"Damn straight," another chimed in, licking his lips. "This is a once-in-a-lifetime chance to fuck a tight, young cunt."

"Exactly," I replied, feeling my pussy throb at their crude words. "So make the most of it. Be rough, be wild—I can take it, trust me."

"Shit, this is gonna be one hell of a week," a third man remarked, his eyes roaming over my body hungrily.

"Speaking of our last night together," I continued, drawing their attention back to the information I was sharing, "let's talk about rule number four." They waited with bated breath as I explained, "Every man who fulfills his commitment to feeding me three daily semen meals will earn the right to join the ass-banging group on our final night before departure. I'll be outside, tied up somewhere, and you can all take turns pounding my tight little asshole as much and as often as you want."

"Jesus Christ," one man gasped, shaking his head in disbelief. "You're really serious about this, aren't you? I wasn't sure on the video call."

"Absolutely," I replied, relishing the excitement coursing through my veins. "I want you all to use me, abuse me, and make me feel like a fuck doll, a sex object."

"Your ass is gonna be so sore after we're done with it," another man laughed, his eyes filled with lust.

"Bring it on," I challenged, my eyes narrowing seductively. "I can't wait to feel your hard cocks slamming into me, stretching me out, making me scream. But for now, boys, here's the fifth rule: the dive resort has assigned a dive boat just for our group. Every morning, we'll go out for a 2-tank dive. While on that boat, I will be nude for your viewing pleasure."

The men were immediately salivating at the thought.

"Fuck," one of them muttered under his breath. "You're seriously going to be naked in front of us every day?"

"Absolutely," I confirmed, my nipples hardening at the thought of being so exposed and vulnerable. "I'll put on a wetsuit for the actual dive, but as soon as I'm back on the boat, it comes off."

"Jesus, you're not even gonna wear a bikini?" another man asked, his voice full of disbelief and lust.

"Nope. Completely nude. I want you all to enjoy the sight of my body—my tits, my pussy, everything. And it's not just for looking... You can touch as much as you want," I added, smirking at their reactions. Their cocks were probably all hurting by then, with not enough room in their pants.

"Amazing," one guy breathed, shaking his head in wonder.

"Alright, now for the sixth rule," I continued, my excitement building as I fed off their desire. "On the morning of departure, it'll be Father's Day. And on that day, any man old enough to be my Daddy gets to give me a spanking right there in front of everyone else."

"Are you fucking serious?" one of the older men questioned, his eyes wide with shock and anticipation.

"Dead serious," I replied, biting my bottom lip. "I'll be naked, over your knees, and you can spank me like the bad girl I am. I've no doubt I'll have been very naughty throughout the week, so I'll deserve it, right?"

"Fuck," another man groaned, his eyes glazed over with lust. "I've never spanked a girl before, especially not one as sexy as you."

"Good," I purred, pleased to be introducing them to new experiences. "It's about time you learn how to discipline a naughty little slut like me. And it looks like I'll be in for a real treat when it's time to fly back home. With all the ass-banging and spanking in the last 24 hours, sitting down on that plane might be a bit of a challenge."

"Oh!" one of the men chimed in, smirking. "Seeing you struggle to sit down? That's gonna be amusing as hell."

"Maybe we should take bets on how many bruises you'll have by the end," another man suggested, earning laughs from the group.

"Speaking of bruises, you can do anything you want with my body as long as there are no permanent physical marks. Now, listen up! I've got a couple more rules for you. These are important too."

"Rule number seven," I continued, my voice low and seductive.

"You need to treat me like a fuck doll, sex toy, or piece of meat. Don't hold back—I want you to give in to your darkest, most animalistic urges. Use me, abuse me, share me, do whatever it takes to satisfy those primal desires deep within you."

"Fuck," one man groaned, his eyes darkening with lust. "That's... that's really something, baby doll."

"Exactly," I purred, delighted at their reactions. "I'm not just some pretty face to admire from afar. I'm here for you to use and enjoy, so don't hold back."

"Damn, girl," another man muttered, his gaze traveling up and down my body. "You're really going all out for this trip, aren't you?"

"Of course," I replied, my eyes twinkling with mischief. "That's why we organized this trip, right? I'm not just your ordinary dive instructor, am I?"

The men chuckled, clearly excited by the prospect of having me at their mercy for the entire week. It only served to fuel my own desires, making me crave the rough treatment they would hopefully subject me to.

"Alright, rule number eight," I said, drawing in a deep breath. "As your fuck doll, I must not have orgasms all week." The men stared at me, their eyes widening in surprise. "I only get off from clit stimulation, so just stay clear of caressing it. You can look at my clit, and even pinch it if you want, but don't pleasure me."

"Pinch it?" one man asked incredulously, his eyebrows shooting up. "Wouldn't that hurt?"

"Exactly," I replied with a wicked smile. "It'll hurt, and that will prevent me from having an orgasm. Think of it as vengeance against a clit some wife of yours forced you to eat in the past. This is your chance."

"Fuck," another man chuckled, shaking his head in disbelief. "Get ready for a lot of pinches. Damn fucking clits!"

"Not a fan of giving oral sex to your wife, are you?" I quipped back, feeling my excitement rise at the prospect of being used so roughly. "If any of you make me orgasm, you're disqualified for the ass-banging night."

I had given myself a challenge to not have an orgasm for the entire year in order to prove that I was nothing but a sex object, and I didn't want that trip in June to derail me.

"Rule number nine," I continued, my voice dripping with desire. "You need to unleash your primal, bestial sexual urges this week. Do things you've never done before—and may never have the chance to do again. Use me, share me, abuse me, and be rough."

"Any specific examples?" a man asked, his eyes gleaming with anticipation.

"Think along the lines of... choking me while you're pounding me, using me as a footrest while someone fucks my face, or tying me up and having a bunch of take turns on my body like it's some kind of carnival ride." The men let out low groans, their eyes darkening with lust as they imagined the possibilities.

"Are you sure about that?" Theo asked, raising an eyebrow as he looked me up and down.

"Absolutely," I insisted. "I want to be the cure for emasculation. Grab me by my hair and force your cocks deep into my mouth. Don't worry if I choke or cry; that's what I crave. Can you make a chick cry?"

"By the way, I can take it all in, but if you want to truly maximize the pleasure, grasp my head and push it downwards until my top lip is resting against your belly and my bottom lip is pressed against your balls. Hold me firmly there until I tap your leg. I can be your deep-throat toy!"

"Damn," Ralph muttered, his eyes fixated on my half-naked boobs. He licked his lips, envisioning the possibilities.

"Or how about bending me over and pounding my tight little ass without mercy? Can you beat my ass into submission? Listen to me scream while you claim ownership of my flesh," I continued, my voice dripping with lust.

"Fuck, Delisha," Fred exclaimed, gripping his crotch in desperation. "You're making it hard to wait."

"Well, do you guys have any ideas?" I asked, eager to know how these men envisioned using and abusing my body. Their eyes sparkled with lust as they began to share their twisted fantasies.

"Maybe we could take turns shoving our cocks in your mouth while you're tied up helplessly," Cliff chimed in, his hand instinctively adjusting the bulge in his pants. "You won't be able to scream or beg for mercy."

"Sounds perfect," I agreed, my pussy throbbing at the idea of being completely at their mercy, choking on thick rods that were gods to me.

"Ever had a man slap your tits, Delisha?" Theo asked, eyeing my perky breasts hungrily. "I bet they'd bounce beautifully under the force of a strong hand."

"Those pretty blue eyes of yours would look even better with tears streaming down your face as we force you to gag on our cocks," Charles observed, still analyzing what I had said earlier, his voice rough with desire.

"Maybe one of us should sit on your face, smothering you with our balls while the others take turns fucking your wet cunt," Edgar suggested, licking his lips in anticipation.

"So you guys think you are man enough to beat my pussy into submission?" I replied, feeling my arousal reach new heights.

"Alright, Delisha," Fred started, looking at me with a hint of concern. "But how will we know if we've gone too far?"

"Lotus. It's my safe word. If I say it, you stop immediately. But come on, boys," I taunted them playfully as we continued our crude conversation at the airport gate. "I don't believe you're capable of pushing me to use my safe word. Every guy I've ever dared to get me there always ended up holding back."

"Really? You think we're just like all those other men?" Francis asked, a slight smirk playing on his lips.

"From my experience, yes. You all talk big about abusing a young chick, but when it comes down to it, you get gentle and gentlemanly. It's like you forget that I want it." I rolled my eyes, feeling frustrated with their caution.

"Is that a dare?" Albert questioned, raising an eyebrow.

"Damn right, it is!" I exclaimed, excitement coursing through my veins. "So here's an idea: let's see if any of you can actually make me use my safe word before this scuba & sex week is over."

"Interesting," David mused, scratching at his beard. "And what happens to the guys who make you beg for mercy?"

"Good question," I replied, tapping a finger against my chin. The wheels in my head turned rapidly as I tried to think of a suitable reward for the men who could prove me wrong. "How about... the first one who gets me to say 'Lotus' wins something? We'll have to brainstorm some options, though."

"Maybe they get to pick the position and location where you'll be fucked next?" Harvey offered, eagerness flashing in his eyes.

"Or choose the type of kinky activity we try out?" Fred suggested, a hint of mischief glinting in his gaze.

"Those are all great ideas," I mused, "but we need to come up with something that really raises the stakes. Something that'll truly motivate you."

I looked around at the eager faces of the 14 men surrounding me, their eyes filled with lust and determination. The stakes had been raised; I could feel the intensity in the air, and for once, I thought perhaps these men would really use my body as much as I wanted them to.

Suddenly, a brilliant idea came to me. My heart raced as I spoke up, wondering if I would regret it.

"Alright, guys, how about this? The first one to make me use my safe word gets an entire week with me as their personal sex slave in Miami. You'd have to fly down at your own expense, but you can stay with me at the beach condo and do whatever you want to me for a whole week."

The men's eyes widened, and I could practically see their cocks hardening inside their pants. They exchanged excited glances, their raw desire evident as they began to talk amongst themselves.

"Fuck, that sounds amazing," Stanley said, licking his lips hungrily. "Just imagine a full week of using her tight little body however I want. Alone, without all of you monkeys! But could we fly you somewhere else instead?"

"Sure," I immediately answered, excited by the unknown.

"God, I'd love to tie her up and force her to suck my cock every morning on my boat," Charles chimed in, his eyes locked on my mouth.

"Like I'll do all week, you mean?" I said, smirking.

I felt moistness between my legs, my body aching for their touch and their abuse. Hearing their fantasies fueled my own, and I couldn't wait to be their willing prey. I wanted them to break me, to take ownership of my young female body, and to push me to my limits until I was nothing more than a submissive, brainless fuck doll for their pleasure–a dumb blonde!

"Alright, boys, it's settled," I announced, grinning wickedly. "The first to make me say 'Lotus' will get that week in Miami with me as his sex slave—or wherever you fly me to. Now, let's get back to the last couple of rules."

"Here's the tenth one: you are not allowed to use my real name. That's too friendly and human. No, to remind yourselves that I'm just a fuck doll, a sex toy, a slut, you must dehumanize me, calling me by those names or any other degrading names you can think of." I paused, letting the impact of my words sink in. "Anyone who calls me by my real name will be disqualified from the ass-banging night."

A mix of excitement and shock crossed their faces, but they quickly nodded in agreement. "You got it, whore," one man said, testing out the new language.

"Perfect," I replied, feeling the thrill of being objectified course through my veins. "Now, which two lucky men get to share my body tonight?"

Ralph, the divemaster, checked his list. "Victor and Albert, you're up first."

"Can't wait," Victor grinned while Albert devoured me with his eyes.

"Upon arrival, you boys should check into your cabin while I confirm the nudity arrangements for the dive boat with the general manager. After that, I'll head over to Albert and Victor's cabin, where I expect all 14 cocks to be ready for my first semen meal of the trip." My voice was sultry and assertive, leaving no room for doubt about what I wanted—and what they would give me.

AS WE WAITED FOR BOARDING, I couldn't help but feel the heat building between my legs. The thought of being used and degraded for the pleasure of this group of old men excited me beyond belief.

I have been thinking about an *extreme* 'sex & scuba' week from the first day I dove. I had worshipped many old gods on prior dive trips. I had been used and abused on many dive trips. But I was always looking to bring it up a notch. Would I finally reach my limit? Would I finally use my safe word?

My nipples hardened beneath my thin top as I could sense the men's eyes on me, eager to ravish my body as soon as they had the chance.

THE BOARDING ANNOUNCEMENT echoed through the airport, snapping me back to reality. I turned to the group of cock-carrying beasts, my heart pounding in anticipation. "Alright, boys," I said with a wicked grin, "it's time for us to board. If you want to start using me as a sex toy, feel free to take turns sitting next to me on the plane. For instance, you can check that I'm not wearing any panties."

I could see their eyes light up at the prospect of beginning our week of debauchery ahead of schedule.

As we made our way onto the plane, I noticed the stares from fellow passengers. The combination of my revealing outfit and the hungry gazes of a large group of men surrounding me must have painted quite a picture. I reveled in the attention, feeling my arousal intensify. I was the luckiest girl in that terminal.

Once we settled into our seats, Albert was the first to slide beside me, his eager eyes raking over my body. I glanced around to make sure no flight attendants were watching before grabbing his hand and sliding it down my belly and under my shorts until I felt his fingers on my wet pussy.

"Can't wait to test drive that tight young fuck hole of yours," he whispered, sending shivers down my spine.

"Me too," chimed Victor, sitting on the other side of my middle seat, grinning like a predator eyeing its prey. I felt a thrill knowing they would both have their way with me soon enough.

Throughout the flight, several of the men switched places with each other, taking turns sitting next to me while I worked on this first sex report for you, guys.

Each one found an opportunity to touch me in some way—running their fingers along my collarbone, caressing my inner thigh, or even daring to reach beneath my shorts to finger my pussy or beneath my tank top to pinch my nipples. My body ached with desire; I was already their plaything, and I knew that once we arrived at the resort, all hell would break loose—a special kind of hell that would be paradise to me.

In between their moves, I found myself lost in thoughts of the week to come.

Initially, when I proposed this trip, I simply wanted a week on a sperm-only diet with a large group of men. My goal was to increase the amount of male milk I had consumed in my life, following a conversation started with a fan who was trying to evaluate how much semen I had swallowed in my young life so far. And the idea of doing it during a dive trip was just because I love scuba diving almost as much as I love the taste of semen, especially from old cocks.

But now, my appetite to be brutality used had grown to an insatiable level, demanding to be abused in such a way that would leave these men shattered from carnal pleasure. My loins ached with anticipation as I imagined myself submitting to their every depraved desire.

Yet, anxiety still coursed through me as I sat on the plane. Would this group of men be real men? I ached for them to take me and use my body according to their will—to force upon me cruel sexual acts that would make me feel no more than a mere piece of meat, of no value other than a tool for pleasuring their cocks. My mind raced wildly as I sat there, yearning for the sexual violence these men could easily unleash on my small, young female form if I could convince them that I was serious about it.

I imagined being tied up and used by this group of hungry old wolves, my body a plaything for their twisted desires. I envisioned their rough hands gripping my breasts, slapping my ass, and pinching my clit as they took turns pounding into me while I cried and begged for mercy (but without using my safe word).

"Enjoying yourself, slut?" Ralph asked, sitting down next to me with a smirk. He must have noticed the glazed look in my eyes as I daydreamed about the debauchery that awaited us.

"Can't wait to be abused," I admitted, my voice barely more than a breathy whisper. "I want you all to take out your darkest fantasies on me."

"Be careful what you wish for, whore," he warned, his hand slipping under my shorts to give my pussy an inspection. "You might just get it."

UPON LANDING, I went to see the general manager of the resort with whom I had exchanged emails to plan our "special" trip. He was eager to get our business because dive resorts had been hit hard by the pandemic. Via video call, he agreed to let our group use a dedicated dive boat for a two-tank dive every morning, and he was committed to assigning a captain and a divemaster who would be fine with me being naked on every boat ride.

That's what I thought we had agreed on.

But once I met with him at the resort, I had a stunning surprise. He had understood that I wanted to be naked for the whole week, all over the resort. He had already notified the staff, and he had sent a message to the other divers booked at his resort for that week. The message explained that there would be a young social media influencer doing research about public nudity for a school paper. Wow!

I was thrilled, as I am sure you would have expected! However, he asked me to wait until Sunday afternoon to be nude because he had some divers leaving Sunday morning, and the new group who had been notified of the nudity project was arriving during the day on Sunday. The resort was not sold out. Besides our group of 14, there would be another 17 divers, and the cool thing was... All of them were men, he said! That was no surprise to me because scuba diving is still mostly a male baby boomer activity, which is one of the reasons I enjoy it!

After the meeting with the general manager, I met our group to feed on their 14 cocks for my first meal. Afterward, I showed them the sex toys I had brought in my backpack, and then I slept in the first cabin to have my body for a full night.

Unfortunately, it wasn't an exciting night. The two men in the cabin used me one after the other, never the two of them together. And the sex was pretty vanilla, using only my pussy since I was wearing a butt plug and they both had enjoyed a blowjob minutes earlier.

On Sunday morning, I showed up for breakfast in my bikini, ready for another 14 loads of male proteins, but it didn't work out.

There was just not enough time to suck 14 cocks before the early morning dive boat departure.

I was drinking water at a table with Harvey when I voiced my sadness and concern about how the trip had started. None of them seemed inspired by the sex toys and restraints I had brought. The first night of sex had been very boring. And now I wasn't getting my sperm breakfast.

Harvey suggested I feed on their cocks on the dive boat on the way to the dive site. I liked the idea. And then he promised to spice things up for me if I agreed to trust him.

I was more than happy to give him my body.

And he sure delivered!

PHASE II
The First Day

4

Forcefully Stripped & Held Down by Old Men on a Dive Boat

The sun had barely risen on the first day of our week-long dive trip as I stepped onto the dive boat, feeling the warmth of its rays caressing my skin. The black material of my bikini contrasted sharply with the vibrant orange trim, drawing attention to my firm breasts and the curve of my hips. My long blonde hair flowed freely down my back, swaying gently with each movement.

The contrast between my youthful sensuality and the aged appearances of the 14 old men in my group was striking. I felt their eyes roving over my exposed flesh, and a thrill ran through me. I wanted them to see me, to desire me, to objectify me. Their hunger for my body only fueled my own depraved desires.

"Morning, boys," I purred, my voice dripping with seduction, as I bent over to drop my dive gear, giving them a perfect view of my round, pert ass.

I had chosen the black and orange bikini today instead of wearing it on Day 3 as originally planned because it was the least revealing outfit I'd bought for the week. Since most of these men had never seen me naked, I wanted them to yearn for what lay beneath the fabric, to build up their anticipation for when they'd finally witness my young firm breasts and smooth, bald pussy. Every other piece of clothing in my backpack was transparent or barely covering anything.

Their lewd comments filled the air, making my nipples harden beneath the thin fabric of my bikini top. "Damn, girl! You're a walking wet dream!" one of the men called out, his voice rough with lust.

I smirked, knowing full well the effect I had on old men. They were like hounds, salivating at the sight of fresh meat. And I reveled in it, the intoxicating power of being the center of their raw, animalistic desires.

"Careful now, boys," I teased, biting my lip and winking at them. "Wouldn't want to get too excited before our first dive, would we?"

"Fuck the dive," growled Theo, his eyes locked on my bouncing tits as I moved about the boat. "I'd rather dive into that tight pussy of yours, girl."

A chorus of agreement and crude comments erupted from the other men, their words like gasoline on the fire of my arousal.

Theo was no stranger to my sensual games. He had been on a dive trip with me when I was an eighteen-year-old new dive instructor, along with Fred, Harvey, and nineteen other men who weren't on this current trip. Today, he looked at me with that same possessive hunger I remembered from six years ago.

"Come on, boys!" Harvey yelled to the other thirteen old men while grabbing my arm. "Let's help ourselves to a taste of our beautiful fuck toy here."

In a surge of playful adrenaline, I managed to free my arm from Harvey's grasp and leaped off the boat, landing back on the dock with a thud. I didn't dare look back as I bolted away from the dive boat, my heart pounding in my chest.

I ran along the rough wooden planks of the dock, dodging scuba diving gear and cylinders that littered my path. My mind raced, torn between fear and exhilaration. The thought of being pursued like prey by these depraved old men sent shivers down my spine, igniting a primal desire deep within me to be their sex object, used and shared at their whim.

"Get back here, you little cock tease!" I heard Harvey shout behind me, followed by the pounding footsteps of the men giving chase. Their crude laughter filled the air, urging one another on as they hunted me down.

"Remember how featherweight she was when we stripped her naked on that trip years ago?" Theo called out, his voice dripping with lustful memories. "She deserves a good beating for making our cocks wait this long!"

As I rounded a corner, I could hear Fred panting heavily, barking commands to the other men. "Corner her! Don't let her get away!"

I knew I couldn't keep running forever, but the thrill of the chase fueled my every step. An inferno of desire burned within me, stoked by their crass words and fervent pursuit. I wanted them to catch me, to dominate me, to force me into submission, and make me their plaything.

My legs felt like jelly as I stumbled over a coil of rope, nearly losing my balance. Gritting my teeth, I pushed onward, determined to draw out this primal dance for as long as I could.

"Look at her juicy ass bouncing as she runs!" yelled one of the men, his voice filled with dark anticipation. "I can't wait to sink my cock into that tight little hole!"

"Her bouncing tits are driving me wild!" another chimed in, his voice thick with desire.

Their vulgar comments only served to motivate me, my body coursing with lustful energy. I wanted them to catch me, to strip me down and devour every inch of my young, nubile body, to be reduced to nothing more than an object for their twisted pleasure.

Suddenly, a forceful grip yanked at my long blonde hair, sending searing pain through my scalp as it pulled me back. My body collided with one of the men, his hard muscles pressing against my soft flesh. My breath hitched as my conflicting emotions surged – fear mingled with an intense desire to be stripped naked and used by these ravenous beasts.

"Gotcha, you little cock tease!" he growled into my ear, his hot breath fanning across my skin. "You think you can run away from us? You're gonna pay for that."

As I struggled against him, the other men closed in, their eyes wild with lust and anticipation. They grabbed my arms and legs, their hands like steel vices around my limbs, causing the blood to rush to my fingers and toes as they lifted me.

I squirmed and writhed, feigning distress while secretly craving the feeling of being utterly powerless and objectified.

"Please, don't hurt me!" I cried out, playing my role to perfection. "I'm sorry! I didn't mean to run!"

"Too late now, sweetheart," a man snarled, his face twisted in a sinister grin.

"Look at her squirm," one man sneered, his eyes fixed on my belly. "She's just begging for it, isn't she? Wants us to strip her down and fuck her raw!"

Their crude words only served to fan the flames of my desire, and I fought harder against their grip, knowing full well the futility of my struggle. I wanted them to tear off my clothes, to expose my naked flesh to their ravenous gazes, and to use me as they saw fit.

"Once we get her back on that boat, boys, she won't know what hit her," Harvey barked, his eyes raking over my barely-covered form hungrily. "Remember that trip when she was just 18? We stripped her down and made her squirm, but we never got to taste that sweet pussy. We won't let that happen this time around, will we?"

"Damn right," Theo chimed in, his grip on my wrist tightening painfully. "I've been dreaming about fucking her ever since. She made us all hard, now it's time for her to pay."

"Please, don't do this," I cried out, my acting skills in full force as I pretended to be terrified.

They dragged me violently along the dock, my body swinging back and forth as four men held me by my ankles and wrists. I felt like a lamb being hauled to a slaughterhouse – a small piece of meat next to these men. The men laughed and taunted me with crude remarks about what they intended to do to me.

"Can't wait to see how much this little cock tease can take," one man sneered, gripping my wrist tighter.

"Maybe we should tie her up and take turns pounding that tight little pussy of hers," another chimed in, licking his lips as he eyed my body.

I yelled and begged for mercy. "Please, don't do this to me!" I cried out, struggling against their grip.

But my pleas fell on deaf ears. They continued making vulgar comments about my body and the extreme sexual violence they had in store for me. My heart raced with a mix of fear, humiliation, and excitement.

These men saw me as nothing but a cock tease who deserved a violent beating, just like I told them to do at the airport the day before. I was just not expecting them to actually act on it. Men readily talk a big game but often turn out to be gentle even when I tell them not to be. Could it be that this trip would give me what I wanted?

"Let's see how much this pretty little blonde can handle," one man growled, his gaze fixated on my exposed flesh. "I bet she'll scream real nice when we start pounding her."

"Nothing like teaching a cock tease a lesson, eh?" another chimed in, tightening his grip on my ankle. "We should take turns using her every hole before our first dive – make sure she knows her place."

"Please, don't do this! I beg you!" I cried out as I struggled to break free from their hold. But they simply enjoyed holding me as a captured animal. All they could see was a young, vulnerable blonde who deserved a beating for arousing their deepest desires.

Back on the dive boat, Harvey barked orders at the other men to strip me naked. As the captain steered us away from the dock, I felt the last shred of safety vanishing into the distance. My young body, firm breasts, and flowing blonde hair seemed to awaken the men's primal lust as if I were an irresistible candy.

"Let's get that top off," Harvey commanded, a sinister grin spreading across his face.

With rough, eager hands, they removed my bikini top, exposing my young, firm breasts to the leering gazes of the old men. Only three of them had seen me in the nude when I was 18 years old. For the other 11 old men, my young female body was something to discover, and their crude laughter filled the air as they commented on my nakedness.

"Damn, look at those tits! Just begging to be played with, ain't they?" one man jeered. Another added, "I can't wait to see how hard those nipples get when we're pounding the cunt."

"Wow! Haven't seen young tits like that in years... Fuck! Decades! Before that chick was born, probably!"

All the while, I yelled, cried, and fought to free myself, but their grip remained unyielding. They stripped me of my dignity as much as they stripped me of my clothes. I realized I had asked them to play rough with me, but nevertheless, I was stunned by how much these old men really saw me as nothing more than... I don't know! A piece of art, a sculpture to unwrap for their twisted pleasure. And how much a young girl's nude body was desirable for these men who could all be my Daddy.

"Time to lose the bottoms too," one of the men growled, his eyes filled with lust. My heart raced as they yanked my bikini bottom off, not caring about the pain it caused me. The rough fabric scraped against my tender skin, leaving a burning sensation in its wake.

"Look at that sweet young pussy; bet it's tight as fuck," someone snickered. Their crude laughter echoed around me as I struggled, and for the first time, tears streamed down my face, probably from a mix of pain and joy.

"Can't wait to see how it feels wrapped around my cock."

"You know she's younger than my two daughters?"

"Don't think like that, man; she's no daughter; she's a naughty cock tease," Harvey chimed in. "Now the bitch's gonna pay for it."

My naked body trembled as I fought against their hold, but it was no use. The more I writhed and pleaded, the more excited they became. It was as if my fear and vulnerability only served to fuel their perverse desires. It was a very unique, raw, bestial scene.

They dragged me over to the bench in the middle of the boat, my naked flesh pressed hard against the rough, unforgiving surface. Each man holding my limbs tightened his grip, forcing me down onto my back. I whimpered in pain, feeling utterly exposed and helpless.

"Get her nice and spread out, boys. Let's give everyone a good look," Harvey barked, clearly enjoying his role as the ringleader of this twisted spectacle.

"Make sure you really hold her down," one of them advised while sneering at me. "This little cock tease deserves every bit of what's coming to her."

The men were brutal in their handling of my delicate, powerless body. They forced my legs apart, giving the entire group an unobstructed view of my smooth, hairless pussy. I could feel their hot, hungry gazes on my most intimate parts, starting with my vulva's outer lips, and it made my skin crawl.

"Please, don't do this!" I cried out, but the men were too consumed by their own depravity to care about my suffering.

"Shut up, slut," one of them snarled as they continued to manhandle me. "You brought this on yourself."

My arms ached as one of the men gripped my wrists tightly, forcing them above my head. My back arched involuntarily, thrusting my young, firm breasts toward the leering faces surrounding me. The crude jokes and laughter intensified as the men ogled my body like ravenous beasts.

"Look at those tits, boys! They're just begging to be played with!" Harvey cackled, his eyes locked on my chest. "She's a cock tease, alright. Maybe we should keep her tied down all week. Teach her some manners."

"Please, don't hurt me!" I sobbed, struggling against their hold. I felt exposed and vulnerable, knowing all eyes were now fixated on my nude tits and bald, glistening pussy.

"Bet that tight little cunt hasn't had a real man yet," another chimed in, licking his lips. "Just begging to be stuffed with a real man's cock!"

"Fuck! I haven't seen such a young girl naked in... Forever!" one man suggested, his grin malicious and predatory that gave me shivers. I love it when I provide old men with pleasure they have not or rarely experienced.

"Young? I've never seen a cute girl like this before. I mean... besides Playboy! Fuck! We get to fuck a Playmate!"

Those words made me forget all the pain. I was proud of my body. I spend a lot of time working out and grooming my body to be attractive to men. So, I always appreciate it when my efforts pay off.

The intense emotions coursing through me threatened to overwhelm my senses. Fear, humiliation, and helplessness clashed inside me, amplifying my desperation while mixing with joy at seeing these old men appreciate the young, nude female body they held in their claws.

I also knew I would be publishing and sharing this sexual experience with you guys, and knowing your cocks would also get hard motivated me even more.

"Please, don't do this!" I screamed, tears streaming down my face again from joy and pride.

"Shut up, you little slut! You had fun teasing us, and now it's our turn to have some fun. You deserve every bit of this," Harvey growled, his voice dripping with menace.

Harvey was the reason this group of men didn't return to a gentlemanly attitude. He was the fuel that made this trip extreme and memorable.

"Look at those perky tits," one man jeered, his voice a lecherous growl. "Just beggin' to be slapped and squeezed!"

"More like pinched and twisted," another chimed in, snickering. "She's just a dirty girl who needs to learn her place."

The more they held my nude body captive, the more violent their comments became, giving me shivers.

"Damn right. We should keep her on a leash, make her our fuckin' pet," a third suggested, his eyes roving over my naked body as if he were choosing furniture.

"Imagine her crawling around like a dog, ass up in the air, mouth open for our cocks," someone else added, saliva practically dripping from his lips.

"Please, stop!" I begged them, tears continuing to stream down my face. "I didn't mean to tease you! Just let me go!"

"Shut up!" Harvey barked, grabbing a fistful of my hair and yanking it back. "You wanted this, you filthy cock tease!"

"Look at that sweet little mouth of hers," one man said, smirking as he stared at my parted lips. "Perfect for stuffing with a hard dick."

"Or her long neck... perfect for choking while we fuck her hard," another added, making choking gestures with his hands.

"Those tender nipples are just asking to be bitten," another man laughed, his eyes zeroing in on my trembling breasts. "I'd love to sink my teeth into them."

"Like hell you would," another man challenged. "I want to twist them till she squeals!"

"Such a flat belly," remarked another, running his gaze along the curve of my stomach. "Perfect for splashing cum all over."

"Please, I don't want this!" I sobbed, my voice breaking as I continued to struggle against their grip. "Why are you hurting me?"

"A good life is for good girls," Harvey sneered. "You're nothing but a naughty, filthy girl who needs to be taught good manners... and respect for the elders!"

"Exactly," someone else agreed. "Her cunt'll be so wrecked by the time we're through, she won't be able to walk." The laughter that followed was harsh and cruel.

"Maybe we ought to see how many fingers we can shove up that tight pussy of hers?" one man suggested, winking lewdly as he held out his hand.

"Better yet, let's see how many cocks she can take at once," another said, his tone almost gleeful. "I bet she'd just love being stuffed full of dicks."

"More like begging for it," someone else interjected. "She's probably never been truly satisfied."

"Look at her squirming," someone else laughed. "It's like she loves it!"

"Of course she does," another replied, his voice oozing contempt. "She's nothing but a fuck doll who was born to be used by real men."

"Please... please stop..." I pleaded, my voice barely audible over the chorus of degrading remarks and crude jokes.

"Sorry, sweetheart," Harvey drawled, his eyes glittering with dark amusement. "You brought this on yourself. Now you're going to get exactly what you deserve."

And I couldn't wait!

5

14 Old Men Took Ownership of My Clit & Used It To Punish Me For Being a Cock Tease

My heart pounded rapidly in my chest as I felt the rough hands of one of the men push aside my outer lips and hood, exposing my clitoris to the leering gaze of the other men on the boat. All I could do was struggle and whimper, trying futilely to escape their grasp.

"Would you look at that?" the man holding my pussy open exclaimed, his voice dripping with crude humor. "I bet she's never had a real man play with her clit before."

"Probably only used those pathetic little vibrators," another chimed in, laughing heartily. "She won't know what hit her when we're done with her."

"Maybe we should take turns flicking it, see how much she can handle," suggested another man, his eyes gleaming with perverse delight.

The room filled with laughter, and I could feel my face burning with humiliation. I had unleashed evil when I encouraged them to be rough!

“No orgasm,” I yelled. I was much more concerned about keeping my commitment to not having an orgasm for a full year than about any pain these beasts could inflict on the dumb blonde.

Following that reminder, without warning, Harvey reached down and pinched my exposed clitoris, digging his nails in it and pulling on it forcefully. Pain ripped through me, and I couldn't help but let out a guttural scream that seemed to echo off the dive cylinders on each side of the dive boat. It wasn't an act anymore. My body twisted in agony, but there was no escaping the cruel grip on my sensitive flesh.

"Ha! Listen to that!" Harvey crowed, obviously pleased with himself. "She really does like it rough, doesn't she?"

"Keep going, buddy," another encouraged, a cruel smile on his face. "Let's see how loud she can get."

Harvey pinched and pulled my clitoris again, sending another wave of searing pain through me. I couldn't help but scream once more, tears streaming down my face – tears of pain this time. As I fought against the men who held me captive, they seemed to feed off my pain and distress, their laughter growing louder and more raucous with each cry I made.

"Look at her," one of them jeered. "She's begging for more!"

"Maybe we should just keep doing this until she passes out," another suggested, his voice dark and sinister. "That'll teach her not to tease men."

"NO!" I wailed, shaking with terror and misery. My tears streamed down my face like a waterfall as pain and fear flooded through me. The men simply laughed, oblivious to my suffering. By then, to these men, I was nothing more than a plaything to be used for their sickening pleasure. My body was just young flesh to be experimented upon by a gang of evil cock-carrying beasts. As nails at the end of another thumb and forefinger took hold of my clitoris, I wondered how much I could bear in this week-long ordeal.

Yet, I had no intention of using my safe word. These men were doing what I had asked them to do when we met at Miami airport.

The pain from my clitoris being pinched and pulled only intensified as another man reached out, his rough fingers grabbing hold of my sensitive flesh. He twisted it without letting go, causing me to yell in extreme pain, tears now streaming down continuously on my cheeks. I couldn't believe how merciless these men were, treating me like a doll to be tortured for no reason but their evil amusement.

"Ha! Look at her squirm! She's really feeling that, isn't she?" one of the men taunted, their laughter ringing in my ears as they egged the cruel man on. "Twist it more, man; let's see if she can handle it!"

As the man continued to twist and pinch my clit, I fought desperately against the grip of the men holding my ankles and wrists down, but it was no use. The pain was unbearable, yet somehow, these monsters found it entertaining. And I wanted more of it!

The man's wicked grin widened as he uttered the words, "Hey, blondie." His dripping fingers pinched my clit with increasing force, his nails digging in to ensure he kept his grip, and I let out an anguished scream. Tears surged and released uncontrollably from my eyes, and I begged quietly through spasms of pain, "Please... stop..."

But each cry for mercy was met with a harder pinch until I thought my flesh would tear from the pressure.

"Is this what you wanted when you teased us at the airport yesterday?" he purred mockingly.

My body felt like it was on fire, yet I kept whispering pleadingly for him to stop. Then came his cruelest taunt yet; "Aw, come on now. You have to admit, you're enjoying this just a little bit, aren't you? Or a whole lot, maybe?"

The wave of pain that washed over me seemed unbearable, and although it made me ill to do so, my lips parted, and I heard myself whisper in submission, "Yes... I love it." His laughter rippled coldly across my skin as he held his nails and his painful grip on the most sensual and private part of my body.

"Good girl," he smirked, not easing up on the pressure. "Now, thank me for giving you what you deserve."

"Thank you," I choked out, pretending to hate myself for saying it.

"See, boys?" the man boasted to his comrades. "She loves it. Our little slut is finally learning her role his society!"

And it wasn't the end of it.

"Who's next?" one of them called out. "Come on, don't be shy! Our little cock tease here deserves it!"

The pain was relentless, each new tormentor vying to outdo the last as they took turns torturing my clitoris while other men kept holding my wrists and ankles down against the hard bench. My screams echoed through the ocean, but there was no one to hear them – no one who cared, at least.

In fact, the men's excitement grew as they observed my torment, their lewd laughter filling the air louder each time I yelled from agonizing pain as if my voice and theirs were a sickening symphony. One after the other, they lined up to take their turn with my aching clitoris, each bringing his own brand of sadistic pleasure to the mix. As my body eventually convulsed almost continuously in agony, I could feel their eyes hungrily devouring my naked form.

"Make her nipples hurt too!" one man shouted, prompting several others to reach for my breasts and twist and pull at my nipples until they throbbed in pain alongside my abused clit.

Despite the excruciating sensation, I couldn't help but find some twisted satisfaction in being so thoroughly used.

Tears streamed down my face, real tears of pain, but I refused to beg for mercy anymore. I reminded myself that I had asked these men to be rough with me and that I wouldn't use my safe word unless absolutely necessary.

The truth was that men who were truly willing to abuse me like this were rare, and I intended to savor every brutal moment.

I clung to consciousness as the searing agony wracked my body, gritting my teeth against the shrieks of pain that ripped from my throat. I convulsed like an animal in a trap, desperate and primal.

At the same time, I thought about telling my Mom and Dad the story of this extreme sexual experience. My Mom, in particular, had always pushed me towards risks, claiming such things would help me explore and discover my deepest sexual needs. This was just another thrilling page in the novel of my life as a sexually liberated woman.

"Look at her, boys," one man boasted while yanking on my swollen clit. "She's not even begging us to stop anymore. Our little cock tease is finally learning to enjoy her punishment!"

"Damn right!" another chimed in, gripping my nipple tightly between his fingers. "She's becoming the perfect fuck toy... pain slut... she was meant to be!"

The crude comments only stoked my determination to endure the torture. I had sought this out, after all – the raw, primal hunger of these men driven by their uncontrollable lust for a young blonde female body. It was an intoxicating mix of pain and pleasure that I wasn't sure when I would get to experience again.

"Who's next?" one man asked, his voice heavy with determination, like a torturer on a mission. "Don't be shy – for once, you don't need to pleasure or lick the clit! Just give that clit a beating!"

As more men gathered around to inflict their own brand of sadistic pleasure upon my vulnerable young body, I embraced the pain, knowing that it would bring me closer to understanding the very depths of my own desires. And as the boat rocked beneath us, as if carrying us further into an evil abyss, I couldn't help but feel a perverse thrill at what awaited me in the darkness.

I was a lucky girl. I've always been.

6

Fuck The Rules! Fuck The Girl!

My body quivered as I lay naked, helplessly pinned down on the bench in the middle of the dive boat. The fourteen men in our group surrounded me, their eyes filled with a primal hunger for the vulnerable young girl flesh in front of them. They took turns torturing my clit and nipples, each twist and pinch sending excruciating pain rippling through my body.

I could hear their laughter as they reveled in my pain, finding entertainment in my suffering. My mind began to numb from the agony, but I refused to use my safe word – this was exactly what I asked the old men to do at the beginning of our week-long dive vacation, to use and abuse me by unlocking their wildest primal instincts. My cries and screams disappeared over the ocean, but I wasn't asking them to let me go anymore. I wanted more.

One man, his fingers rough and calloused, pinched my burning clit mercilessly while another twisted my already beaten nipple between his thumb and forefinger. "You like that, don't you, slut?" he growled, his breath hot against my earlobe. In response, a shameful moan escaped my lips.

"More," I begged, wanting to push the limits of my own

endurance. The men exchanged glances before continuing their violent exploration of the young, vulnerable female body they kept captive, each tormenting touch driving me further into a world where pain and pleasure melded together.

As I writhed beneath their cruel hands, my thoughts swirled with the perverse realization that I had become nothing more than a 20-something female body for them to vent their anger against all cock teases they had ever encountered.

I didn't care. Actually, I did. It fueled my desire for degradation. I wanted them to use me, break me, tame me, own me – anything to satiate their bestial lusts.

"Please," I whimpered, real tears of pain streaking down my cheeks as the relentless torment continued. I was exactly where I belonged – in a life of submission and debasement at the hands of twisted, pervert old men. And at that moment, despite all the pain – or maybe because of it – I wouldn't have traded it for anything.

Harvey, the ringleader of this twisted game, spoke up with his voice dripping in lust.

"Fuck the rules," he spat, his face contorted with desire. "Theo! You've waited six years to feel her tight cunt wrapped around your cock. Are you gonna wait another three days?"

He motioned to the two men at my ankles, who eagerly spread my legs even wider, keeping my pussy exposed and vulnerable. I could feel the heat of their gazes between my thighs as Theo dropped his bathing suit, revealing his hard, pulsating cock.

Without a moment's hesitation, he plunged into me, the force of his thrust making my breath catch in my throat. The sensation of being filled by him – of seeing him finally take what he'd been denied for so long – was intoxicating. This old cock had wanted to fuck me for six years since a previous dive trip. Me. My body. My pussy. I was a special girl!

By the way, as I mentioned before, conversations in these sex confessions have been abridged to make it flow easier for you, and well... Because my memory is not perfect, especially when I am aroused!

"See how you like this, you little cock tease!" Theo growled, his eyes wild with lust as he pounded into my aching core. The more he fucked me, the deeper he went, stretching my walls to their limit.

"You're going to be his fuck doll all week, Delisha... I mean, cunt," Harvey snarled, his hand gripping my hair tightly. "Every part of your tight young body is going to serve him. And everybody. Got it?"

As Harvey coached Theo to claim me, I couldn't help but revel in the degradation. I had wanted this – needed it – and now I was getting exactly what I had craved.

"Please," I whispered, my voice choked with arousal. "Use me. Make me yours."

"Damn right, I will," Theo replied, his pace never faltering as he continued to drive his hard rod into my tight pussy. His words stoked something dark within me, and I felt myself spiraling further into submission, every brutal thrust pushing me closer to the edge.

"Remember, whore," he hissed, sweat beading on his brow as he loomed over me. "This is what you deserve for being such a fucking tease."

My body ached from the relentless pounding Theo delivered to my tender, vulnerable pussy. As he continued his assault, two men held my legs wide open, stretching me painfully. The others looked on, some with concern.

"Is this okay?" one asked hesitantly. "This wasn't part of thc plan for this week."

Fred chimed in, reminding them of my own words. "The dumb blonde wanted us to abuse her, remember? She even dared us to push her to use her safe word. If the little cunt wants a beating, who are we to deny her?"

Their faces shifted as they nodded in agreement, like sheep. I couldn't help but feel a twisted thrill at their animalistic determination to dominate me.

"You're right!" one of them eventually declared. "Fuck all the rules! Fuck the girl instead!"

Theo grunted, sweat dripping down his face and onto my belly as he fucked me mercilessly, his cock fighting my butt plug for real estate inside my body. "God, your tight little pussy feels amazing," he growled. "You've been teasing me with this sweet hole for six years, and now you're going to pay – with interest – all week!"

Tears streamed down my cheeks, mainly from the burning pain in my clit, but I didn't want him to stop. I wanted to be their plaything, their sex pet. The crude names they used to describe me only fueled my desire for more.

"Look at this perfect fuck toy," said one man, his rough hands pinching my nipples hard enough to make me cry out even more. "We're going to beat you into submission, baby girl. By the time we're done with you, you'll be begging."

"Please," I whispered through gritted teeth, trying to find some semblance of control in the midst of my torment.

"Quiet, slut!" Harvey snapped, slapping my face. "You are not allowed to come this week. It's the only rule we'll respect!"

Their malicious laughter echoed in my ears like a chorus of evil, taunting me with the threat of being used without ever experiencing the pleasure of climaxing. Little did they know I hadn't experienced an orgasm since the year had started, and I relished in that pain. The more men take advantage of my body, the more I feel as though all of my essence has been sucked away – leaving me an empty sex doll to be exploited for their own selfish desires. That feeling of craving, yet being deprived of fulfillment, is exactly what I yearn for, binding me with chains of endless anguish.

"Remember, Miss Dive Instructor," Theo hissed, his grip tightening on my hips. "You asked for this. You wanted us to treat you like a worthless fuck toy."

I nodded as the truth of his words sank in. This was what I had craved, what I had begged for. And now, there was no turning back.

"Thank you," I whispered, my voice barely audible over the sounds of their grunts and laughter. "Thank you for giving me what I deserve."

Theo finally pulled out of me, his cock slick with my juices. I barely had a chance to catch my breath when Fred stepped forward, a predatory gleam in his eyes. Gripping my hips, he positioned himself between my legs and thrust into me without warning. My body involuntarily tensed at the sudden invasion, but a moan escaped my lips as he filled me completely.

"God, Delisha!" Fred growled, his voice strained with lust. "I've been wanting this tight little cunt for so long... You have no idea what you've done to us all these years."

As Fred began to fuck me hard, the other men continued their assault on my nipples, pinching and twisting them mercilessly. The pain was excruciating, but it only fueled the fire raging within me.

"Tell me," Fred demanded, his thrusts growing more forceful, "tell me that you deserve this. That you're nothing but a naughty girl who needs to be taught a lesson."

"Y-yes," I stammered, struggling to find words through the haze of pain and pleasure. "I deserve this... I'm a naughty girl."

"Damn right, you are," Fred snarled, his grip on my hips tightening. "Now, say you need to be taught a lesson like the little evil babe you are."

"I... I need to be taught a lesson," I confessed, my cheeks burning with humiliation. "Please... punish me."

A wicked smile spread across Fred's face as he slammed into me even harder, driving me closer to the edge. But fortunately, before I could reach climax, he pulled out and stepped back, leaving me empty and aching.

"Who's next?" Fred asked, smirking at the group of older men waiting eagerly nearby.

David didn't waste any time taking Fred's place. As soon as his cock was inside me, he started pounding me with a ferocity that left me breathless. His hands moved to my breasts, slapping them roughly as he growled.

The other men continued their assault on my nipples, their laughter and crude comments echoing in my ears as they reveled in seeing my body twitch in pain with my arms still stretched above my head and held down by strong beast hands. My emotions were a whirlwind, a tumultuous mix of pain, humiliation, and an overwhelming desire to be used by these perverted old men just like I'd always wanted – just like they deserved, I even thought, wondering how married sex had been for them.

With each thrust, each slap, and each cruel taunt, I felt myself being pushed further into submission. And as much as it hurt, as much as it debased me, I couldn't deny the thrill that coursed through me at the thought of being at their mercy, completely and utterly lost to their depraved desires like a prey held down by hyenas feasting on soft flesh.

David finally finished with me, his groans of satisfaction echoing in my ears as he pulled out. I barely had a moment to catch my breath before the next man took his place between my legs. He grinned wickedly at me, excitement clear in his eyes as he positioned himself.

"Always wanted to fuck a perfect '10'," he growled as he thrust into me, filling me with his hard length. "A beautiful babe like you... but don't think it'll make this any easier on you, slut."

As he forced his hard cock inside me, the other men resumed their wretched assault on my nipples. Every time they pinched or twisted them, I writhed in agony, yet with every new wave of pain came an unexpected pleasure racing through me. I couldn't believe that I was actually experiencing this torture and humiliation, just as I always liked but so rarely got. They were treating me like an object, a toy for them to play with, a living being in a laboratory of horror, and the more they did it, the more I wanted it.

The man fucking me leaned down, whispering filthy things in my ear as he pounded my tight cunt mercilessly. "You like this, don't you? You love being our little cock sleeve for the week."

I could barely think straight from the overwhelming mix of pain and pleasure, but I knew he was right. This was the reason I organized this dive trip in the first place. And now that I had it, I was desperate for more. Well, actually, I had organized the trip with the simple goal of drinking an overdose of sperm all week, but... This was better. Much better!

He was soon replaced by another eager old man who had been waiting his turn to abuse the young, nude blonde girl.

"I've always wanted to feel the tight pussy of a young Playmate! God, you're beautiful!"

His words. Not mine!

But then the boat captain spoke up, his voice tinged with admiration. "It sure is a beautiful sight, watching you boys tame a young blonde slut," he said, his eyes trained on me as I lay there, panting and spent. "I'd love to have a run at her myself, but we've reached the dive site. If you want to dive, it's now or never. Sex or no sex, we have to be back at the dock for noon."

The men who hadn't had their chance with me grumbled in disappointment, but Harvey had more twisted ideas to please everybody.

7

14 Old Men Savagely Beat My Clit To Force Me To Agree I Didn't Deserve To Go Scuba Diving

Harvey asked the captain for a rope and quickly tied my hands together, then forced me to stand beneath a metal bar in the canopy of the boat. With another swift motion, he secured the rope, leaving me dangling there, my arms stretched above my head.

"Let's see how you like this, little pet," he snarled, stepping back to admire his handiwork. "Maybe it'll teach you some obedience."

I struggled against my restraints, feeling strangely more vulnerable and exposed than before. My arms ached above my head, stretched and bound to the metal bar, forcing me to stand right there in the middle of the area where divers gear up. My clit and nipples throbbed from the relentless abuse they'd endured, but even as pain coursed through me, I couldn't help but yearn for the depths of the ocean.

I love scuba diving almost as much as I love worshipping old cocks.

"Please," I begged, my voice strained from crying. "Let me go diving with you. I'll do anything you want; just let me go down there."

"Shut up, cunt," one man snarled. "Toys don't talk back."

"Come on, guys," I persisted, desperation clawing at me. "I promise I'll make it worth your while."

"You'll make it worth our while?" Harvey growled. "We don't need you for that. We'll use your body to make our trip worth its while!"

My clit and nipples throbbed in agony, but the desire to go scuba diving burned within me. I was standing on bare feet, utterly naked, with my arms above my head and wrists bound to a metal bar on the roof of the dive boat. Through gritted teeth, I kept begging the 14 old men surrounding me to let me go diving with them.

Scuba diving is an intense passion, second only to being used by old men.

"Shut up," one of them snarled in response, "sex toys don't talk back, we said."

But I couldn't help myself. The urge to dive was overwhelming, so I kept begging. Harvey, the ringleader, decided he'd had enough and reached for my tenderized clit to teach me another painful lesson. Instinctively, I moved away as far as the rope binding my wrists would allow. The old men laughed, amused by my futile attempt to escape their cruel intentions.

"Look at her," one of them sneered, "trying to get away like she doesn't know what's coming." Their crude words cut through me, reminding me of my place as their plaything and pain slut.

Harvey's face darkened, and he motioned for the other men to hold me in place. One man stepped behind me, gripping my waist tightly, but as Harvey reached for my clitoris, I instinctively fought to keep my legs closed.

"Keep her legs open!" Harvey barked, his voice rough with excitement. Two men grabbed my thighs, their fingers digging into my tender flesh as they forced my juicy, young legs apart. I struggled in vain, my body writhing against their harsh grip.

"Teach this little slut a lesson, Harv!" one of the old men shouted, his eyes gleaming with lustful anticipation.

"Make her beg for our cocks instead of begging to dive!" another chimed in, his words dripping with depravity.

"Show her she's nothing but a set of holes for us to use and abuse —all week," said yet another, the sinister undertone sending shivers down my spine.

My clit already throbbed with pain, and my heart raced as I realized that my desire to scuba dive was overshadowed by these men's hunger to humiliate and own me. Their crude language painted an explicit picture of how they saw me—a helpless, beautiful babe put on earth for their pleasure.

"Finger pinching her clit doesn't seem to have taught her anything," a voice observed.

Harvey smirked, clearly enjoying my torment. Encouraged by other men to find a stronger way to teach me to be submissive and obedient, he dug through his dive gear and brandished a large black binder clip that he removed from an underwater slate, waving it in front of my face like a sadistic magician. With a twisted grin, he snapped the metal ears of the clamp open and closed, making me flinch each time the jaws clamped shut.

"Think you deserve a more serious lesson, little bitch?" he taunted, the malice in his voice palpable.

My breath hitched as I stared at the menacing binder clip, my mind racing with images of the excruciating pain it would inflict on my sensitive clit. The fear churned in my stomach, mingling with the adrenaline pumping through my veins. Part of me wanted to scream my safe word for them to stop, while another part craved the degradation and control they exerted over me. I was getting more than I had hoped for, and it was just Day One!

"Go on, Harvey," one man urged. "She needs to know her place."

"Come on, Harv," another man egged him on as I squirmed in place. "She deserves it. Show her how a real man handles a slut like her."

"Besides, she has a safe word if it gets too much," another chimed in, his eyes gleaming with perverse anticipation.

I didn't want to use my safe word. I knew I would share this sexual experience with you guys, and knowing your cocks would get hard motivated me to push my limits.

"Make sure she never forgets that her only purpose is to be our fuck doll," added one more, rubbing his hands together eagerly.

My heart pounded in my chest as the men unanimously encouraged Harvey to take things further. They were treating me like a piece of meat for their amusement, and yet, I couldn't shake the thrill that coursed through me.

"Alright then," Harvey said, finally relenting to the pressure. He nodded at one of the men, who quickly moved to spread my outer lips apart. My clit hood was pushed aside, exposing my vulnerable clit to the cool air, making me shudder.

"Look at that pretty little thing," Harvey smirked, holding the binder clip open and inching it closer. The metal looked cold and unforgiving.

"Here we go," he whispered just before the jaws clamped down on my clit. The pain was immediate and excruciating, like nothing I had ever felt before. It tore through me, forcing a scream from my throat.

The old men gazed with eagerness at my tormented form, their lips stretching into menacing snarls as they relished every moment of my torture. I could feel the searing agony emanating from my clamped clitoris and flooding through every inch of me, its intensity amplifying with each relentless heartbeat. Desperate to assuage the pain, my toes curled in agony, my anus clenched tight, my body trembled uncontrollably, and tears streamed down my face. The sheer brutality of these men was astonishing, and as I hung there, my body convulsing in pain, I realized I should have used my safe word, but I still didn't want to. I can be a brat like that!

There was something intoxicating about being at the center of their twisted desires—and it terrified me that I loved it so much!

"Look at her twitch! That's what you get for teasing us, you cock-hungry slut!" one of them jeered, while others laughed and continued to make crude comments about my body.

My legs gave way, but the men holding my thighs moved to hold me in suspension in mid-air by grabbing my ankles, preventing at the same time my body from convulsing as much as it wanted to. As I hung there, the old men laughed and came closer to inspect the damage they had inflicted upon me.

"Look at that cute little clit suffer," one man sneered. "It's about time a pretty blonde like her gets a taste of her own medicine."

"Damn right!" another agreed. "I can't tell you how many times I've been turned down by girls like her. Now, she knows what it feels like to be the one begging."

"Her clit probably doesn't even know what hit it," a third man chimed in, his voice dripping with sadistic glee. "Just imagine all the times she's teased it with those slutty fingers of hers. Now, it's getting what it deserves."

As they continued to mock me and my aching clitoris, I couldn't help but remember my prior clit torturing sessions. At the time, I thought I had reached the maximum pain I could tolerate. But none of it compared to this—the sheer intensity of the pain, the humiliation, the desperation I felt as these men reveled in my suffering.

"God, I hate eating my wife out," one man suddenly confessed, his face contorted with disgust. "Seeing a clit take a beating like this is oddly satisfying."

"Ha! Yeah, my ex never let me anywhere near her pussy for years," another added. "Well, look at me now, bitch. I'm watching this sexy young thing get torn apart while you sit at home, alone and miserable."

Their laughter and crude comments stung me, but at the same time, a twisted part of me reveled in their attention. I had asked for this, after all. I had challenged them to use me to vent out their anger against prior clits and women, and they were doing just that.

"Remember," one man said, his voice dripping with menace,

"this is only the beginning. You've got a whole week with us, and we're going to make sure you never forget it."

"We'll make sure *we* never forget it!" Harvey clarified.

The burning pain in my clit intensified as Harvey pulled on the rubber band attached to the paperclip. My body trembled, and tears streamed down my face. I couldn't help but let out desperate pleas.

"Please... please," I cried, while the pain was almost unbearable.

"Say it," Harvey growled, tugging the rubber band harder. "You don't deserve to dive because you're nothing but a naughty cock tease."

"Please," I begged, but the men around me only grinned, urging Harvey on.

"Come on, slut," one of them taunted. "Admit that you're just a sex pet, and pets don't dive."

My body shook uncontrollably from the pain, and I finally choked out the words. "I... I don't deserve to dive... I'm just a sex pet... Pets don't dive."

"Look at her squirm!" one of them barked. "She's just a brainless fuck doll, and her needs mean nothing!"

"Never seen anything so beautiful in my life," another added, his eyes glued to my tormented naked body by then covered with my tears flowing down between my tits and onto my belly on their way to the clamp at the source of them.

Finally, after what felt like an eternity, Harvey removed the binder paperclip from my swollen clit. The sudden rush of blood back into the sensitive flesh sent my body shaking even more violently than before. The men's laughter grew louder, their dirty comments and violent remarks echoing in my ears.

"Bet she's never been used like this before," one of them sneered. "Just look at her shake—she can't handle it!"

"Can't wait to see what else we can do to her," another said, his eyes filled with a dark hunger. "This is so hot."

My body still trembled from the intense pain, tears streaming down my face. Some of the old men stared at me with a sick fascination, their eyes filled with hunger.

"God, look at her cry," one of them muttered, licking his lips. "There's nothing more beautiful than watching a dumb blonde babe like her break down."

"Right?" another man agreed, his eyes wide with excitement. "The way her body shakes with her tits bouncing... fucking incredible."

More of the old men chimed in, their crude comments and perverse admiration fueling their desire for more of my suffering. I could feel their eyes roaming over every inch of my naked, vulnerable form.

"Come on, Harvey," one of them urged. "She's so damn sexy. Let's see more wobbling young boobs."

"Teach her a lesson she won't forget for the rest of the week... or more," another added, smirking.

With a nod, some of the men approached me, their hands reaching out to caress my trembling body. They wiped away my tears as if they cared for me while their words painted a different picture.

"Sweetheart, you need to learn your place," one of them whispered into my ear. "You'll thank us later when you realize how much better it is to be obedient."

One man held my cheeks in his rough hands and kissed me on the mouth. "You're so fuckin' hot, babe!"

"Such a pretty little thing," another murmured, his fingers picking up tears between my young firm tits. "But you have to understand that this is what you were made for—to please and serve real men."

Their twisted affection gave me shivers, but there was a part of me that couldn't deny the thrill I felt at being so completely dominated by these old men. They had broken me down, exposing my rawest, most primal desires.

"Look at her cry," one man chuckled darkly, his voice dripping with perverse excitement. "There's something so fucking beautiful about a young blonde babe like Delisha sobbing and shaking like that."

"Damn right," another agreed, his eyes glued to my naked form as if I were the most captivating thing he'd ever seen. "I've never seen anything so arousing in my life."

"Please," I whimpered, trying to maintain some shred of dignity. "I've learned my lesson. Just let me go diving with you."

"Damn! Harv! She didn't learn her lesson!"

"Aw, poor thing," Harvey taunted, a cruel grin stretching across his face as he held the binder clip menacingly in front of me. "You want more, don't you, sweetheart?"

"NO!" I screamed at the top of my lungs as he clamped the unforgiving metal down on my sensitive clit once more. My body convulsed violently, the pain searing through every nerve ending.

"Fuck yes!" one of the men roared with laughter, seemingly intoxicated by the sight of my suffering. "That's what she gets for being such a cock tease!"

"Make her beg, Harvey!" another urged him on, his excitement palpable as he watched the scene unfold before him.

"Alright, bitch," Harvey growled, gripping the rubber band attached to the binder clip and yanking it, sending fresh waves of unbearable agony through my tortured clit. "You're going to promise not to ask for anything for the rest of the week, understand?"

"YES!" I cried out, willing to say anything to make the pain stop immediately.

"Good girl," he smirked. "Now tell us that you won't speak anymore unless someone asks you to or you're answering a question."

"Y-yes," I stammered, my voice barely audible over the sound of my own ragged breaths. "I won't speak unless... unless someone asks me to... or I'm answering a question."

"See, boys?" one of the old men cooed, his fingers gently wiping tears going down my flat belly as if he were trying to comfort me.

"She's learning her place. And she'll thank us for it later, won't you, babe?"

"Y-yes," I whispered, allowing the hot tears to continue streaming down my naked body. The thought that they found my weakness and pain so beautiful was absolutely terrifying, yet at the same time, it ignited a spark deep within me that craved their cruel dominance.

"Please," I gasped through my tears, desperation clawing at my chest. "No more."

"Let her cry all week if she wants," another man commented with a lecherous grin. "There's just something so damn irresistible about seeing a perfect-10 Playmate like her in such agony."

I considered again using my safe words, but my stubborn determination held me back. I am known to be stubborn! And then, the captain spoke up, providing me with a timely rescue. "It's a beautiful sight to see a blonde babe cry and twist like that," he said, his eyes devouring my naked, tortured form. "But we'd better get on with the diving."

With a reluctant sigh, Harvey removed the paper clip from my clit for the second time. My body shook in agony as the blood flow returned to the swollen, sensitive flesh. The crude comments of the men echoed around me, each one relishing the sight of my pain and humiliation.

"Damn, I've never seen a woman's cunt take such a beating," one man laughed. "Bet she'll think twice before teasing us... anybody... again."

As the men geared up for their dive, I remained in my stand-up position, naked, with my arms tied above my head. And I couldn't stop the tears from falling. I was missing out on the very thing I loved almost as much as serving the old cocks of these men. Yet, at the same time, I couldn't help but feel a twisted sense of pride that they had unleashed their animalistic instincts upon me, just as I had asked them to do at the airport.

With a mix of envy and longing, I watched the men dive into the water, leaving me on the boat with the divemaster and captain. In my vulnerable state, I found myself wondering if my mother had ever experienced such intense pain in her own clit, or if my father had ever participated in torturing a woman's clit in this way.

I knew it was a strange thought to have, but at that moment, all I wanted was to connect with my parents and share this raw, brutal experience with them. They had always been so accepting of my wild side, and the idea of discussing my most recent humiliation with them only fueled the fire burning within me.

And while the pain was still scorching between my legs, I chuckled. For the first time in my life, I would not be diving during a tropical dive trip in paradise! So much for being a dive instructor! And I would never look at a black binder paperclip in the same way. Think of me when you see one!

8

Old Men Find a New Way To Enjoy a Surface Interval: Spit-roasting My Nude, Young Female Body

I stood naked, hands bound above me, a rope biting into my wrists as the dive boat rocked gently beneath me. My body exposed and vulnerable, I was a lamb awaiting slaughter by the old men who had just plunged into the depths below. The sea's salty breeze kissed my skin, teasing my nipples into taut peaks.

Part of me reveled in this predicament, feeling like a piece of meat for their enjoyment, while another part of me ached to join them underwater. Scuba diving has been my passion since I was 14. And I became an instructor at 18 because I craved that connection with the ocean. Now, my two worlds collided – my submissive desires and my love for the sea.

The captain and divemaster were preoccupied, scanning the horizon for bubbles and other boats. I was alone and ignored, torn between yearning for the old men's rough hands on my body and the urge to be submerged in the depths of the ocean.

AS A FEW OF the old men climbed back on board, I struggled to keep my composure. The water dripping off their gear splashed down onto my feet, each salty droplet a cruel reminder that I had missed out on the dive.

"Look at that," one of them said, grinning as he eyed my naked body. "Our little slut's still here, waiting for us. Look at all that cum dripping from her tight little cunt."

"Damn right," another added, chuckling as he removed his mask. "Can't wait to add mine to the mix."

"Shame she can't join us underwater, though," a third man said, smirking at me. "Oh, right! She's getting a well-deserved cock tease punishment!"

As more of the men returned, their lewd comments grew in intensity. I couldn't help but feel myself growing hot under their vulgar and explicit remarks; a part of me reveled in it, even as my heart ached for the freedom of the sea.

"Bet you wish you went diving with us, don't you?" one man taunted, seeing the longing in my eyes. "Well, tough luck, sweetheart. This week is payback time for you!"

"This week," he said. I thought they would let me dive eventually. But wait! Could they be cruel enough to keep me tied on the boat all week?

As they continued to strip off their gear and ogle my exposed young girl's body, I knew that soon enough, I would once again be at their mercy, satisfying their most primal urges as they used my body to satiate their lust.

"Damn, just look at that fine piece of ass," one man said, his eyes glued to my naked form as he stepped on board. "Never thought I'd see such a perfect fuck doll waiting for me after a dive."

"Shit, you're right," another chimed in, smirking lewdly. "And look at those tits, just begging to be squeezed and slapped. And what a tight little pussy she has."

"Can't forget about that pretty slut face," another added, pointing toward my flushed cheeks. "Just imagine her looking up at you with those innocent blue eyes while she sucks you off. Fuck, this is gonna be the best dive trip ever!"

As they continued to make crude remarks about my body, I couldn't help but feel a twisted sense of pride – these men were completely consumed with desire for me. Me! My body.

Genetics gave me firm boobs, blonde hair, and blue eyes. But I work out to keep my belly flat and my thighs strong. I watch what I eat to keep my waist thin. I work hard for my body to be the way men like it. And it felt good to hear men appreciating it.

"Boys, we should bring her along on every trip from now on," one man suggested. "No more boring surface intervals – just endless hours of fucking this hot little plaything."

"Damn right," agreed another. "Imagine how many other guys would sign up for our trips if they knew they'd have a willing cum dumpster like Delisha here to use and abuse whenever they wanted. I'm surprised there are only 14 of us. Imagine 50 men defiling her all week!"

"Plus, just think about all the different ways we could degrade her," someone else chimed in, grinning wickedly. "We could tie her up, spank her, choke her... Hell, the possibilities are endless."

"Surely beats sitting around, waiting for the next dive," a man in the background quipped, clearly excited by the prospect.

My body, exposed and vulnerable, drew the hungry gazes of every man climbing onboard after their dive.

"Look at that perfect mouth," one man said, licking his lips. "Those plump lips just begging to be wrapped around our cocks."

"Her tits are heaven," another chimed in, his eyes locked on my chest. "Just the right size."

Their crude comments only escalated as they scrutinized my body while removing their dive gear, leaving no part untouched by their lewd words. They spoke about my long blonde hair, remarking how it would make an excellent handle while fucking me; my slender neck, which they imagined wrapped in their grip as they choked me into submission; my flat belly, a canvas upon which they could spill their cum as a trophy of their conquest.

"Those thighs, though," a man said, almost reverently. "Imagine them wrapped around your waist as you plunge deep inside her."

"And don't get me started on her feet," someone else chimed in. "Sexy little toes perfect for sucking on while we take turns ruining her tight cunt."

As men removed their wetsuits to expose a series of big beer bellies, they gathered around me, their hands roaming my naked flesh like explorers claiming new territory. Fingers tangled in my hair, palms caressed my breasts, and rough hands traveled along my back, tracing the curve of my spine. It was as if they were trying to absorb the essence of my body through touch alone.

"Such a sweet, tender piece of ass," one man whispered into my ear as he stroked my cheek. The way he looked at me – with such raw hunger and desire – sent shivers down my spine.

"Can't wait to use and abuse you, babe," another gruff voice said from behind me, his hand gripping my hip so tightly I could feel the marks forming on my skin.

As they continued to touch and grope me, I couldn't deny that their rough affections made my body ache for more.

Surrounded by these old men, I felt like a living sculpture, an object of pure desire – god's gift to old men. And right on cue, one of them, apparently the poet in the group, his eyes gleaming with lust, began to describe my body as if it were a priceless work of art.

"Look at her," he said in a low, sultry voice, "that luxurious blonde hair cascading down her back, framing that angelic face... And those lips, so full and inviting, just begging to be kissed or wrapped around a hard cock."

The other men listened, nodding and murmuring their agreement as he continued, "Her neck, so delicate, strong hands could shatter it, yet strong enough to hold up that lovely head, leading down to those stunning breasts. God, those firm tits with those perky nipples just waiting to be squeezed and contorted... again and again!"

I shivered in pleasure, feeling both exposed and wanted as he went on, "And that flat belly, taunting us with that sensual little belly button, which draws our gaze down lower, to the part we all crave the most: those inviting thighs, leading to the treasure between her legs – that young, tight pussy."

"Let's not forget those seductive feet," another man chimed in, "with 'spermivore' written on her toes. She has an insatiable hunger for our seed, guys!"

I wondered how many women never got to experience the exhilaration of being a naked, vulnerable, desirable piece of meat among a group of male beasts. From my teenage years, I've always believed young women should explore their sexuality with old men before settling down, getting married, or whatever.

I want to be ravished, beaten, and abused by groups of old men for a few more years before I consider a steady boyfriend and marriage with a boy my age. Old men crave young chicks, and it would be selfish of me not to satisfy them. I do not understand girls who don't jump on this opportunity. They are missing out on intense thrills.

"Talking of spermivore," one man suddenly exclaimed, "We're supposed to feed this sperm-hungry chick three times a day, and we haven't done it yet!"

Hands grabbed me, pulling me in different directions until a burly man untied the rope holding my arms up, forced me on my knees, and shoved his cock into my eager mouth.

"Feeding time!"

Meanwhile, another gripped my hips and thrust himself into my dripping pussy from behind.

"Fuck her up, dude! Pound that tight little cunt!" one man shouted, egging the two men fucking me. "Choke her with that cock! Make her take it all!"

"Rip her apart!" another man barked, his words dripping with lust and aggression.

I reveled in their vulgar cheers, my body aching for the brutal treatment they were so eager to give. The animalistic way they saw me only added fuel to my desire to be used and abused by these men - to let them use my body to please god, which for me, is an old man's cock.

As they took turns ravaging my mouth and pussy, their crude words echoing in my ears, I knew I was exactly where I wanted to be – at the mercy of their bestial hunger for sex and violence. Vanilla sex was just not for me.

My body quivered as the men took turns pounding my pussy and forcing their cocks down my throat, one after the other. Their voices were harsh and brutal, encouraging each other with extremely violent language.

"Make her choke on it!" one man growled, his eyes wild with lust.

"Ravage that tight cunt, tear her apart!" another snarled.

The sound of their crude words filled the air. I was nothing more than an object they owned, and I craved every moment of it.

"Fuckin' slut deserves this," a man sneered, gripping my blonde hair tightly as he slammed his cock into my mouth.

"Damn right she does; look at her taking it like a whore," another agreed, thrusting himself deep inside my dripping pussy from behind.

"Good-looking bitches like her always act like cock teases," one man spat. "She's just lucky we're here to put her in her place."

"Blondes like her are practically begging for a beating," another added, smirking as he gazed at my exposed body.

After an hour of being spit-roasted by the ravenous men, my body ached and trembled with exhaustion. Then, the captain's voice rang out, announcing the beginning of the second dive. His words were like a cruel reminder of what I was missing out on – the underwater world that I loved so dearly.

"Hey, bitch," one man grunted, delivering a stinging slap to my ass, "We ain't done with you yet."

"Such a shame you won't be joining us for the dive," another taunted with a wicked grin. "The first one was incredible, and we expect the second to be just as beautiful." Their laughter echoed in my ears, torturing me with the knowledge that I wouldn't be able to experience the underwater paradise they spoke of.

I was on a dive boat on a dive trip in a tropical paradise, and I wasn't allowed to dive!

I yearned to join them, to escape this relentless torment. But then, the memory of Harvey's sadistic treatment of my clit surged back into my mind. The lingering pain in my sensitive bud reminded me that asking to go diving had only resulted in more suffering. And so, I resigned myself to my role as their submissive sex slave.

"Can't have it all, can you, slut?" one of the men sneered, reading my conflicted expression. "Somebody had to teach you a lesson one day, right? Fuckin' cock tease!"

"Maybe after we're done using you, we'll let you lick the salt off our balls," another added, his eyes gleaming with sadistic amusement.

Harvey tied my hands behind my back and told me to remain on my knees until they returned. I obeyed. Just like that.

AS THE SECOND DIVE ENDED, the men returned to the boat with satisfied grins plastered across their leathery faces. I remained on my knees, hands still tied behind my back, as I watched the cum that trickled down my thighs, mixing with the saltwater caressing my knees. The crude laughter of the men filled the air as they took in the sight of me, my body glowing with sweat and semen.

"Look at that drippin' cunt," one of them sneered. "You're just like a fuckin' leaky faucet, aren't you?"

"Can't wait to add my load to that mess," another chimed in, his swollen cock already straining against his swim trunks.

My pussy throbbed at their words, yet my heart ached for the underwater world I had missed out on. As if sensing my inner turmoil, one man pressed his dripping mask to my cheek, smirking as he said, "Too bad you couldn't join us, but it's punishment time for you... all week."

"Get ready for round two, bitch," a gruff voice declared, and soon enough, I found myself being spit-roasted once again. My mouth stretched wide around a thick cock, while another slammed into my wet, abused cunt from behind.

"Fuck her hard, boys, make her feel it," someone shouted, urging them on as they pounded me relentlessly. My abs burned as I strained to keep myself at 90 degrees, my bound hands preventing me from getting support from my arms. I was on all fours but with only 2 support points!

Between the thrusts on my ass and choking on cock, my mind wandered to the ocean I longed for, imagining the vibrant marine life that danced just beneath the surface. It was a cruel irony – my passion for the ocean was now tainted by my submission to these old men.

"Make her choke on that dick," a man barked, gripping my hair tightly as his friend rammed his cock further down my throat. I choked, incapable of breathing, tears streaming down my face as they continued to use me for their pleasure.

"Make sure she doesn't forget her place," another voice chimed in, followed by a sharp smack to my ass. The sting sent shivers up my spine, but this spit-roasting session provided a reprieve from the relentless focus on my clit. For now, it seemed they had forgotten how much they enjoyed torturing my sensitive nub.

"Harder! Fuck her like the worthless cum dumpster she is," someone shouted, inciting more laughter and cruel encouragement from the others.

As I endured this brutal treatment, a part of me craved the

roughness, the objectification. I was torn between the desire to be abused and the longing to be free, exploring the depths of the ocean I loved so dearly.

"Harder," I managed to gasp around the cock filling my mouth, embracing the darkness within me even as my heart ached for the underwater world I was denied access to by old men who had claimed ownership of my body for the week.

9

Old Cocks Spit-Roasted My Young Body In Front of Strangers & Made Me Their Dive Gear Slave

As the dive boat sliced through the waves, making its way back to shore, I felt a pang of disappointment deep in my gut. The old men had made sure I didn't get to dive today, punishing me for all the sexy cock tease girls they had met in their lives – especially the blonde ones. I was on my knees again with my hands still tied tightly behind my back, my naked body on display for everyone to see and use.

"Look at you, Delisha," Harvey sneered, his wrinkled hand gripping my waist as he pounded into my young juicy pussy from behind. "How does it feel to be a cock tease, now?"

"Ex-cock tease," Theo corrected, shoving his cock deeper down my throat, cutting off my air supply for at least a minute before allowing me to gasp for breath. "She's now just a cheap slut."

My body quivered under their rough treatment, but a dark part of me craved it. It was an unsettling mix of desire and frustration as I longed to explore the ocean's depths while simultaneously being drawn to worshipping old cocks that were, collectively, my god and my raison d'être.

The boat slowed down, signaling our arrival at the dock. I could hear the captain talking to people on the shore, my face instinctively burning with humiliation as I realized that we would be docking with me still in this compromising position, although, deep down, the exhibitionist in me was overjoyed.

"Give the crowd a good show," Harvey laughed cruelly, slapping my ass hard enough to leave a red mark. "Show them what a dirty slut you are."

"Use her harder," Charles barked at Harvey and Theo. "Really, give those guys something to gawk at."

As the boat came to a stop and was securely tied to the dock, I felt a thrill run down my spine. I knew there were people watching me, witnessing my degradation and abuse. But instead of shrinking away, I found myself eager to please them, sucking on Theo's cock with renewed vigor.

"Look at her go," Stanley chortled, his eyes gleaming with perverse delight. "She's putting on quite the performance."

"Bet she enjoys being our little whore," David chimed in, grinning wickedly.

"Look at those wobbling tits," Harvey sneered, his thrusts growing more forceful as he drove his cock deeper into my tight pussy. "That's what a blonde girl is for."

"Can't get enough of it, can she?" Theo grunted, gripping my head tightly as he rammed his dick further down my throat, making me choke around his girth as he forcefully held my lips against his belly and balls. "Bet she's been dreaming about this moment ever since we first met her."

"Let's give 'em a real show," Charles suggested, a wicked smile playing on his lips. "Don't hold back, boys. Make her scream for everyone to hear just how much she loves being our little cum bucket."

Harvey and Theo took Charles' words to heart, their actions growing rougher, more primal, as they used my body for their own twisted pleasure. I couldn't help but feel a perverse thrill at the thought of so many people watching me like this—exposed, degraded, and utterly shameless in my desire for their approval.

"Harder," I choked out between gasps, my voice muffled by the shaft filling my mouth. "Please... Choke me more."

"Such a greedy little whore," Edgar laughed, slapping my ass hard enough to leave a stinging imprint. "She just can't get enough of our old cocks, can she?"

"Maybe we should invite some of those spectators to join in," Bernard mused, eyeing the growing crowd on the dock with interest. "Really give our cute little Delisha here the full treatment she deserves."

"Fuck yeah," Fred chimed in, the excitement in his voice palpable. "Let's see how much her tight pussy can really take."

Their words spurred on the men currently using me as their personal fuck toy, Harvey and Theo slamming into me with renewed ferocity. I could feel my body ache under their brutal assault, but I didn't care—all that mattered was honoring old men and worshipping their cocks and balls while becoming the ultimate object of their violent, insatiable lust.

"Take it all, you filthy little slut," Harvey growled, gripping my hips tightly as he drove his cock home once more, his climax imminent. "Show these people just how much you love being our plaything."

"Choke on it, you dirty whore," Theo added, forcing my head down until I had swallowed the entire length of his throbbing member, making me choke and splutter as tears streamed down my face. "That's it... you're nothing but a series of holes for us to fill."

The laughter of the other old men rang in my ears as I continued to be violently spit-roasted on the dive boat. The men on the dock had been informed of a nudity experiment by a college girl, but they hadn't expected it to include wild sex. I could hear their shocked and excited murmurs, which only fueled my desire to pleasure the cocks that were relentlessly pounding into me.

"Look at this little whore, getting her holes destroyed," one of the men on the dock called out crudely. "I didn't know that was part of the definition of nudity, huh?"

"Damn," another chimed in. "This cute blonde is putting on quite the show!"

As the strangers watched and commented on my debasement, I couldn't help but feel a surge of energy. It mesmerized me to know that so many people were enjoying being witnesses to my utter submission, and this excitement encouraged me to suck even harder on the cock in my mouth. My throat burned from the relentless thrusts, but I didn't care—all I wanted was to be the perfect plaything for these men.

Eventually, after what felt like an eternity, Harvey and Theo finished using me, their hot, sticky seed coating my throat and dripping from my abused pussy. As I stumbled to my feet, I saw strangers eyeing my naked body with a mix of shock and lust.

Harvey walked over and untied my hands, smirking as he did so. "Alright, Delisha, you are not allowed to dive, but you sure can unload all our dive gear and put it up to dry on those racks," he said, gesturing to the dock.

"Great idea," Bernard added, laughing at me, "it'll be the closest she'll get to scuba diving this week."

I nodded submissively, knowing that I had no choice but to obey. Their words stung, but I knew that this was part of the humiliation I had signed up for—being made to serve these men in every way they desired.

The old men's laughter filled the air as they disembarked from the boat, not bothering to carry any of their dive gear. They had left that task to me, and I knew I wouldn't disappoint them. As I began to unload the scuba diving equipment, feeling the heaviness of the cylinders and the rough texture of the dripping wet wetsuits against my bare skin, my ass welcomed a stinging slap each time I passed one of the old men.

"Move that sweet little ass, babe!" Edgar barked, his hand

making contact with my tender flesh. The other men chimed in, egging him on.

"Make sure she knows her place in society," David added, grinning maliciously.

As I continued my work, I relished glancing at the new faces on the dock. Seven men, likely part of the group the general manager had mentioned earlier, were scrutinizing me intently. Their eyes roamed over my naked body, lingering on my young tits and waxed pussy, drinking in every inch of me as if I were a piece of art on display for their amusement.

"Damn, look at that tight little body," one of them muttered, his voice dripping with lust. "I didn't think we'd get a show like this."

"Can you believe it?" another man said, his eyes locked on my ass as I bent down to pick up another stinky wetsuit. "That's the girl who's gonna be naked all week. Fuck, she's perfect."

My cheeks had a natural reaction of burning with embarrassment, but deep down, I reveled in their attention. It made me feel powerful in a twisted way—knowing that I was the center of their desire, even as I served as a nude dive gear slave.

I focused on the task at hand, trying to ignore the burning pain in my muscles and the constant slaps on my ass. Each time, I gritted my teeth and reminded myself that this was all part of my role as a young girl owned by a group of old men. I was here to satisfy them, no matter the cost.

As I struggled to unload all the scuba diving gear made heavier by being still soaked in seawater, I overheard the manager talking to some of the new men on the dock. "Gentlemen, this is Delisha," he said, gesturing toward me as I bent over to pick up another pair of fins. "She's the one I mentioned who'll be participating in a nude experiment for her college project."

"Damn," one of them whistled, eyeing my exposed body hungrily. "I heard we'd have a naked chick around, but I never expected such a stunning piece of ass." His eyes roamed shamelessly over my curves, lingering on my breasts and between my legs.

"Yeah," another chimed in, smirking at me as I tried to maintain my composure amidst their lewd comments. "I mean, look at those tits—they're fucking perfect. And that pussy... Jesus, it's like she was made for fucking."

Heat spread through my body, a mixture of disgrace and arousal simmering under my skin. Since I started exploring my sexuality as a teenager, I always craved the idea that my body had been designed as a sex machine for men to use. Hearing an old man say it was a blessing to my ears.

As I continued to unload the dive gear, Harvey approached me, grinning wickedly. He reached out and slapped my ass hard, making me cry out in pain and surprise. "Once you're done here, dirty girl, meet us at Victor's cabin," he ordered, his voice low and menacing. "We're going to make sure you're ready for your week as our naked little slave."

I wiped the sweat from my brow as I continued to unload the scuba diving equipment, naked and barefoot on the rough wood of the dock. My arms ached from the weight of the equipment, but I persevered, determined not to give these men any reason to punish me further. I took one heavy item after another off the boat, feeling the sun beating down on my exposed skin and the eyes of the new male divers following my every move.

"Wow," one of them uttered, his gaze locked on my tits as they bounced with each step. "You're really doing all of this completely naked, huh?"

"Yep," I replied breathlessly, trying to maintain my composure as I hoisted another cylinder back to the fill station. "It's part of an experiment for a school project."

"An experiment?" the other man inquired, his eyes roving over my body, lingering on my smooth, bald pussy. "What kind of experiment involves being a naked slave?"

"Long story," I admitted, shifting the weight of the cylinder while trying to protect my naked toes.

"Damn," the first man murmured, shaking his head in disbelief. "Well, I can't say I'm not enjoying the view."

I grinned at him, feeling a surge of pride that even in my current state, I could still make these men weak in the knees with desire. These old men found it erotic to see a young, vulnerable, thoroughly nude chick in a crowd of dressed old men, and strangely enough, I agreed.

As I continued working, two of the male strangers approached me, their eyes fixated on my toes where the word 'spermivore' was painted on my toenails. "So, what does that mean?" one of them asked, curiosity piqued.

"Uh, well," I hesitated for a moment, debating how much to share. "It means I only eat sperm. Semen."

"Really?" the other man's eyes widened, and he looked at me like I was some kind of exotic zoo creature. "That's... wild."

"Yeah," I agreed, feeling a mix of embarrassment and satisfaction at their shocked expressions. "I guess you could say I have a pretty unique diet. But I love it!"

"Can't argue with that," the first man chuckled, his eyes now traveling up my legs, over my toned stomach, and finally lingering on my breasts. "But damn, if it keeps you looking this good, maybe there's something to it. Fuck! Every girl should go on that diet!"

I couldn't help but smile at their blatant admiration, even as I continued to unload the heavy, wet dive gear. As the men stared at me like I was some kind of nude masterpiece, I felt both exposed and empowered—a strange combination that made me crave even more attention.

As I finished unloading the last set of dive gear, I reveled in the knowledge that these strangers had seen every inch of my body from many different angles, and they wanted me. Me! My body. The thought made me feel powerful, desirable, and utterly alive—even if it meant I was still at the mercy of the 14 old men waiting for me at Victor's cabin.

I knew it was time to head to Victor's cabin, as Harvey had

instructed. The thought of what might await me there sent a shiver down my spine, but I couldn't deny the thrill that coursed through me at the prospect of being completely naked and vulnerable in front of so many men at once—all week.

"All week," I kept repeating in my head, ecstatic at the opportunity.

I carefully made my way through the resort, my bare feet occasionally stinging from the rough gravel on the trails. I winced with each painful step, but the discomfort was worth it—the sensation of being completely exposed, every inch of my body on display for anyone who cared to look, was intoxicating.

"Hey there, gorgeous," a man called out as I neared the pool area. I looked over to see him lounging in a deck chair, his eyes locked on my naked young female body. "You must be Delisha, the resident spermivore."

"Oh, you've heard already," I grinned, stopping to chat despite the pain in my feet. My nipples hardened under his gaze, and I could feel the familiar ache between my legs. I loved how strangers can unabashedly stare at my tits, my pussy, my ass—every part of me that society deemed private and off-limits.

I don't understand why nudity is illegal in our prudish, repressive American society. I'm for #FreeTheNipple and #FreeThePussy! But then, I also enjoy that nudity is rare because revealing my intimate female pieces to men who rarely get to see a young girl naked is an indescribable pleasure.

"Got any plans now?" he asked, his eyes lingering on my breasts.

"Actually, I'm meeting some friends at a cabin," I replied coyly, knowing full well that Harvey and the others would have more than just a friendly chat in mind.

"Shame," he sighed, clearly disappointed. "Well, if you ever find yourself with some free time, I'd love to help you with your... unique diet."

"Thanks for the offer," I said, giving him a sultry smile before leaving. "Maybe another time."

As I continued my barefoot journey to Victor's cabin, the feeling of freedom washed over me. It was a stark contrast to the confined spaces of South Florida, where opportunities to be nude were limited to select areas and situations. Here, on this tropical island, surrounded by lush foliage and warm ocean waves, my naked body felt right at home. I couldn't wait to explore every part of this island in the nude—the only one in the nude!

"Damn, I'm one lucky girl," I thought to myself, reveling in the sensation of the gentle breeze brushing against my sensitive nipples and the sun kissing every inch of my exposed flesh. It was exhilarating to be the only one undressed among all these clothed strangers, their lustful gazes devouring me like a tantalizing feast.

The path ahead was a mix of smooth sand and rough gravel, forcing me to adjust my stride accordingly. Each step sent a mixture of pleasure and pain through my body, reminding me of the primal nature of my current state.

By the way, it is not new that I enjoy pain. As a teenager, I liked walking barefoot on gravel – slowly but still. I don't know why. Meanwhile, my best friend thought I was a nutcase. She only tried it once!

"Hey there, beautiful," a man called out from a nearby cabin porch, his eyes locked onto my swaying breasts as I approached. With a coy smile, I greeted him in return, fully aware that my nudity was the center of his attention.

"Hi," I replied, pausing for a moment to give my bare feet a break and to let him drink in the sight of my body before continuing on my way. There is nothing I relish more than pleasuring old men's cocks and delighting their eyes.

The trail led me under the shade of towering palm trees, their fronds rustling gently in the breeze. The sound of the ocean whispered seductively in my ears, accompanied by the calls of tropical birds hidden among the foliage. It was an erotic symphony, perfectly complementing the hedonistic display of my young nude body as I walked.

Every so often, I would encounter another stranger along the path, each one unable to resist stealing glances at my exposed form. Some tried to hide their desires behind a thin veil of politeness, while others were more brazen in their lust. And I loved every single moment of it.

"Enjoying the view?" I asked one gawking old man, arching my back slightly to accentuate the curve of my ass as I passed him. He simply nodded, his eyes glued to my body until I disappeared from his sight.

With each step, I became more and more intoxicated by the knowledge that I was an erotic spectacle for all to see. All week. All over the island. The sun's warm rays caressed my naked skin, and the salty ocean air filled my lungs, reminding me just how alive and free I truly was.

"Is this what paradise feels like?" I wondered, my excitement growing with every footfall, thinking I never wanted to leave.

As I neared Victor's cabin, my heart pounded in anticipation. Harvey's orders had been clear, and I had obeyed without question. Part of me wondered what the group of old men had in store for me when Harvey said they needed to make sure I was ready for a week as their sex slave and nude servant. Another part of me throbbed with excitement at the thought of what lay ahead.

"Ah, fuck," I muttered, feeling a sudden twinge of pain from my abused clit. The beating Harvey had given it earlier as punishment for being a cock tease still lingered, but I had almost forgotten about it amidst the pleasure of walking around the tropical island completely nude. My nipples hardened with each step, and I could feel the heat between my legs growing more intense.

"Guess it's time to find out what these old pervs have planned for me," I whispered to myself, approaching the cabin.

10

14 Cock-Carrying Beasts Used Sex Toys To Reduce Me To a Sex Pet & Establish New Rules For The Week

I arrived at Victor and Albert's cabin, as Harvey had ordered. The air was thick with wanton desire, making the atmosphere heavier than the salty sea breeze that mixed with it. As I walked onto the porch, it felt like a stage set for an erotic spectacle, the ocean waves crashing behind me only adding to the sensual ambiance.

All fourteen old men sat in a circle, their hungry eyes feasting on my nude young body. I noticed Harvey holding my backpack by his feet, a devilish grin on his face. My heart raced, knowing this display of vulnerability thrilled me just as much as it did them. Every inch of my naked flesh was exposed for these sexually depraved old men to devour with their lecherous gazes.

"Go ahead, sit down," Harvey gestured towards an empty chair, but then he stopped me. "Actually, no. Stand right here in the middle of us all. This is where you belong."

Powerless and exposed, my body became a canvas for their lustful imaginations. The men's eyes roamed my curves, drinking in every detail of my nakedness. My nipples hardened under their scrutiny, betraying my own excitement.

As Harvey ordered, I began to caress myself—every inch of my naked body except for my throbbing clit, he said. My fingers traced delicate patterns over my neck, making me shiver. The men's eyes followed my every movement, their lewd comments filling the air with a mixture of adoration and depravity.

"Such a perfect little slut," one man remarked as my hands moved onto my breasts. I squeezed them together, pinching my erect nipples, feeling both humiliated and aroused by their attention.

"God, look at that tight ass," another man groaned when I ran my hands over the curves of my buttocks and down my thighs. Bending over to caress my legs and feet, I knew they had a perfect view of my swollen pussy lips, slick with arousal.

"Can't wait to have those sweet lips wrapped around my cock again," someone else muttered, earning a chorus of agreement from the others.

I stood back up in the center of the circle, heart pounding and cheeks flushed. Harvey opened my backpack and began pulling out my clothes, carelessly tossing them into a nearby garbage can. Panic surged through me as I realized I would be left with nothing to wear for the journey home.

"Please, just let me keep one set of clothes for the flight back," I begged, but Harvey silenced me with a cruel smirk. He held up the black binder paperclip that he'd used earlier on my clit, and my breath caught in my throat, remembering the pain it had caused.

"Remember, you're only allowed to speak when we ask you a question," Harvey warned, his voice low and menacing. "Final warning!"

The sight of the torture device sent a shudder through my body, and I felt the lingering ache in my clit intensify. The men's laughter echoed around me, mocking my helplessness and vulnerability.

"Look at her trembling," one man snickered. "Maybe she actually wants that clamp on her clit."

"Damn," another chimed in. "We're going to have fun with every inch of that gorgeous babe, whether she likes it or not."

As the men continued their crude banter, I felt a perverse thrill at my situation. Despite my fear and humiliation, my body betrayed me, growing even more aroused by the prospect of being used and degraded by these men. The line between pleasure and pain blurred, and I knew that by the end of the week, I would be a completely different person—broken, submissive, and utterly devoted to satisfying their every twisted desire.

Meanwhile, the circle of old men around me continued to gawk at my naked body, their lustful gazes making my skin crawl. I tried to hold my head up high, but the realization that I was completely at their mercy threatened to break my spirit.

"Look what Harvey's got now," Theo said, his voice dripping with excitement as Harvey pulled out my passport, ID, and phone from my backpack. A sickening knot formed in my stomach, my vulnerability reaching new heights.

"Since our little sex pet is just a tamed wild animal now... Theo! Take these and do whatever you want with them. Is there a black market here for passports and IDs? I'm sure you can get something for the phone." Harvey handed my belongings over to Theo, smirking wickedly. The thought of being stranded here without any clothes, means of identification, or communication terrified me, and a sense of panic began to take hold.

"Please... at least let me keep my passport and one set of clothes for the flight back home," I begged, my voice shaking.

"Ah-ah," Harvey scolded, holding up the black binder paper clip that had tormented my clit earlier. "How many final warnings do we give her?"

My heart raced as I stared at the terrifying nightmare device, the pain in my clit a stark reminder of my submission to these men.

"Look at her, begging like the needy little slut she is," one man sneered. "She'll learn soon enough that we own her, head to toe."

"Damn right," another chimed in, licking his lips. "We own every inch of this fine piece of ass, and she better get used to it."

As they taunted me, my mind raced with thoughts of helplessness and fear. But even as I naturally despised them, my body betrayed me, growing more aroused by the degradation and humiliation they heaped upon me.

I discovered a long time ago that I enjoy being nothing but a sex object, and no matter what people think about my sexual practices, they give me great happiness.

"Listen up, sweetheart," Harvey said, his voice cold and cruel. "You're going to be our personal plaything for the rest of the week, whether you like it or not. We control your body, your clothes, your clit, and everything else about you, understand? After that, who cares?"

I nodded silently, my cheeks burning with shame as I accepted my fate. The men around me laughed and jeered, their crude comments only fueling my growing sense of despair.

"Your pretty little face won't get you any special treatment here," one man taunted. "You have holes. We have cocks. Get it?"

"Can't wait to see how much she begs when we're done with her," another added, his eyes raking over my naked form. "By the end of the week, she'll be nothing more than a drooling, moaning mess."

"Damn right," a third agreed, grinning wickedly. "She's gonna learn what it means to be completely and utterly owned by us. I wonder if she will continue to be a cock tease after that."

My heart hammered in my chest as I watched Harvey take out the ankle restraints from my backpack, throwing them at me with a sinister grin. The cold metal landed at my feet, and I hesitated for a moment before bending down to pick them up. The men's eyes roamed over my body as I did so, their lecherous gazes lingering on every curve and crevice.

"Go on, put them on," Harvey barked impatiently. "Show us just how eager you are to be our little fuck toy."

As I wrapped the restraints around my ankles, my fingers trembled with a mixture of fear and excitement. My entire being was consumed by the lustful stares of these depraved men, stripping me of any semblance of dignity or control. Their crude comments echoed in my ears as I secured the second restraint.

"Bet that tight little cunt is already dripping wet, just begging for a good, hard pounding," one man sneered, his voice thick with desire.

With the ankle restraints now firmly in place, Harvey tossed the choker and leash at me next. I caught them in my hands, feeling the weight of the leather and metal against my skin. Desperate to please the men surrounding me, I struggled to fasten the choker around my neck.

"Look at that pretty collar on her neck, like a proper little pet," one of the men remarked, a predatory gleam in his eye. "Just imagine leading her around the dive resort on that leash, parading her naked body for everyone to see... and use."

"Or tying her up outside our cabin so any of us can take a turn whenever we please," another suggested with a wicked grin. "She'll be there, waiting and ready for us, just like the obedient little fuck pet she is."

The leash dangled from my neck, resting between my naked young firm boobs, a constant reminder of my new status as nothing more than a sex pet for these men—a toy for them to use and discard as they saw fit.

Holding the nipple clamps, Harvey smirked. "You know, boys," he said, addressing the group around us, "I couldn't help but notice how much fun you all had watching Delisha scream and squirm when I tortured her clit earlier."

The men around me nodded in agreement, their eyes hungry as they stared at my vulnerable body. One of them licked his lips and said, "Oh, she was a sight to behold, alright. That perfect blonde babe finally got what she deserved for being such a cock tease."

"Damn right," another chimed in. "But I think the black binder clip makes a better punishment than those flimsy clips. More intense, you know?"

Their words stung, but I could feel the heat pooling between my legs at the thought of being punished so severely and savagely on the most sensitive part of my young girl's body. As if sensing my inner turmoil, Harvey grinned wickedly before decisively throwing the nipple clamps in the garbage.

"Alright then, it's settled," he announced. "We'll use the binder clip on her clit whenever she disobeys or steps out of line during this trip." The other men murmured in approval, and I felt a shiver run down my spine at the thought of enduring such pain again. Suddenly, a week seemed like an eternity.

My mind raced with fear and anticipation, trying to process the reality of what lay ahead. I imagined the cold, unforgiving grip of the black binder clip snapping onto my sensitive clit, sending waves of excruciating pain through my entire body. The mere thought made me tremble, yet I couldn't deny the perverse arousal it stirred within me.

Harvey wasted no time, pulling out the dildo ball gag from my backpack. The old men's eyes widened in anticipation as they studied the intimidating 5-inch long dildo penis attached to a strap meant to hold it firmly in my mouth.

"Put it on, Delisha," Cliff commanded, his voice rough and eager. It was clear that these men wanted complete control over every aspect of my body—even my mouth. With trembling hands, I picked up the ball gag and placed the dildo between my lips, adjusting the strap around my head until it was secure.

As soon as the dildo penetrated the back of my throat, I was reminded of its purpose—to keep my mouth and throat ready for their cocks. I struggled to suppress a gag reflex I rarely have, but the relentless length of the dildo forced me to adapt quickly. The men watched intently, grinning with perverse satisfaction as I submitted to their latest humiliation.

"Remember when she thought she could set all the rules for this week? Without even asking our opinion," one of the men snickered, recalling our initial meeting at the Miami airport. "Well, now we make the rules. And we don't need her opinion."

Their laughter filled the air as they began discussing how best to use and degrade me. After some debate, they agreed that I would wear the dildo ball gag at all times, all week unless my mouth were needed to pleasure one of their throbbing cocks.

"Look at her, sucking on that fake cock like a good little slut," one man jeered. "I can't wait to see her choke on the real thing again."

"Yeah, she'll be our personal cocksucker all week long," another added gleefully. "She won't be able to say a word, just like the dumb blonde she is. Either she sucks our cocks, or she sucks the dildo, 24/7."

"Alright, now for the final touch," Harvey said with a twisted grin, pulling handcuffs from my backpack. "We can't have you trying to stop us from enjoying your body now, can we?"

"Her hands should be cuffed all week, too," Charles chimed in, his lewd gaze never leaving my body. "She won't be able to resist us that way."

"Exactly," Harvey agreed, securing the cuffs around my wrists behind my back. I was now utterly helpless, my hands bound, a dildo gag filling my mouth, a butt plug still up my ass from earlier, and my body on full display to these depraved men.

"Look at her," Stanley laughed, eyeing my naked form. "A perfect submissive slut, completely at our mercy. Think she understands *what* she is now?"

"Maybe we should take turns tying her up outside our cabins," Wilfred suggested, his eyes filled with lustful hunger. "That way, we can all enjoy easy access to her tight, young pussy."

"Or better yet, we'll just have her staked out near the beach where she'll be highly visible and available to anyone who wants a go," Victor proposed, eliciting approving nods from the other men.

"Sounds perfect," Albert concurred. "We'll have ourselves a communal fuck doll for the week."

I swallowed hard, my throat already aching from the dildo gag lodged within it. But in the depths of my darkest fantasies, part of me yearned for this utter loss of control, to be used and degraded in ways no woman should ever endure—except me. My Mom always said I had a higher tolerance to pain than anybody she ever knew. And it was not just tolerance. I needed it.

"Let's just make sure she knows her place," Harvey declared, smirking at me. "You're nothing but our sex toy, Delisha. And from now on, the only thing your pretty mouth is good for is sucking cocks... or dildos."

"Having her sleep outside is a perfect idea," Bernard commented, his tongue sliding across his lips. "That way, any one of us can use her whenever we please, day or night."

"Exactly," agreed Charles, grinning wickedly. "We should tie her to a tree or something so she's always available for a good pounding."

Their rules were so much more exciting than mine!

"Let's make sure she's tied up tight, though," Stanley chimed in, his eyes narrowing as they traveled down the length of my bound form. "We wouldn't want our pretty little whore trying to escape now, would we?"

"Of course not," Edgar agreed, a cruel smile playing on his lips. "She needs to understand that she's nothing more than a piece of meat for us to use as we see fit."

"Can you imagine how desperate she'll be after a few nights sleeping on the sand, naked?" Francis mused, his voice dripping with lust.

"Hope it rains," a voice added in a deeply sadistic tone.

"Damn, it will be so beautiful," Victor concurred, his hand stroking the bulge in his pants as he stared at me. "There's nothing like breaking a cute girl's spirit to get her to submit completely."

"Alright then," Harvey declared, a gleam of sadistic delight in his eyes. "It's settled. Delisha, you'll be spending your nights outside, tied up like the wild animal you are. And you better believe we'll be taking full advantage of that."

As I stood there, my heart racing with a terrifying mix of fear and excitement, I knew I had surrendered myself completely to their cruel whims. I had asked them to let their bestial instincts lose, and they were not disappointing me. I craved this ruthless treatment—to be owned and dominated by these powerful, animalistic men who saw me as nothing more than an object for their most vile and violent pleasure.

And we had only been at the resort for 18 hours! Imagine a full week with these beasts... I was a lucky girl!

11

Old Men Savagely Beat My Clit To Train Me as a Sex Slave

I stood naked in the center of the circle, feeling the eyes of 14 old men on my body as they sat comfortably around me. The dildo ball gag filled my mouth, silencing me and leaving me to focus on the sensations of vulnerability that coursed through my veins. I could feel the choker around my neck, a silent threat that any one of them could yank on the attached leash and choke me if they so desired.

My ankles held restraints, not currently attached to anything but ready for use at any moment. My hands were cuffed behind my back, rendering me helpless before these men who feasted their eyes upon my exposed young female body. I could feel the butt plug nestled deep within me, a constant reminder of my status as their plaything.

The eroticism of the situation was palpable. The air around us thrummed with raw, sexual energy. I basked in their stares as they devoured my tits and pussy with their eyes, my exhibitionist nature exploding into a million tiny pieces of pleasure. The old men that surrounded me were wild and thirsty, hungering for what they saw before them—a young, nude, beautiful blonde woman who was willingly submitting to their deepest, darkest desire. The sight ignited an animalistic fervor within each of them, desperate to violently take possession of that young female body.

As I stood there, my body an open invitation to their lustful intentions, I could see the men's arousal growing. Their eyes came back over and over on my perky breasts, the curve of my hips, and the smooth mound between my legs.

At that moment, I was a living piece of art for them to admire, a tantalizing vision of submission and sensuality. They whispered amongst themselves, discussing my predicament and how best to make use of me.

"Look at her," one of the men leaned in close to another, his voice dripping with desire. "She's like a ripe fruit just waiting to be plucked and devoured."

The man beside him nodded, his eyes fixed on the butt plug that filled me. "She's a perfect little sex pet, isn't she? Just imagine all the filthy things we're going to do with her this week."

Bending forward at their command, I spread my legs wide, giving them an unobstructed view of the butt plug nestled between my cheeks and my wet pussy. With every slow turn I made, the men in the circle gasped and murmured appreciatively, savoring the sight of my exposed vulnerability.

"Keep pivoting, just like that," one of the men said, his voice rough with desire. "I want to see every inch of that dumb blonde."

"Fuck, look at that juicy cunt," another man remarked, licking his lips as he stared at the wetness that coated my inner thighs.

As I continued to rotate for their entertainment, I reveled in their lustful gazes, feeling a thrill of exhibitionistic joy surging through me.

"Ah, such a perfect little slut," a third man purred, watching the way my breasts swayed with each movement.

The 14 men began discussing whether my current adornments were enough to make me their true sex pet for the duration of our trip. Their conversation was laced with explicit language and crude descriptions of how they wanted to use and dominate my body.

"Maybe we should add nipple clamps," one man suggested, his eyes locked on my bouncy breasts. "Make her feel that pain while we fuck her like barbarians."

"Or have her wear a tail plug," chimed in another, grinning wickedly. "She'd look so cute crawling around on all fours like a little bitch in heat."

The men's voices grew harsher, their words more vulgar, as they debated whether I had truly grasped my role as their sex pet. My heart pounded in my chest, a mix of fear and anticipation coursing through me.

"Maybe she doesn't fully understand yet," one man suggested, his eyes narrowed as he studied me. "Should we remind her of the consequences? Let her feel that binder paper clip on her clit again?"

A shiver of dread raced down my spine at the mere thought of the painful clip biting into my sensitive flesh once more. I tried to protest, but the dildo gag filling my mouth rendered my pleas unintelligible.

The men laughed at my muffled cries, clearly finding it erotic to see such a beautiful young babe unable to voice her objections, completely at their mercy.

"Look at her squirm," a man remarked, his eyes roaming over my naked body hungrily. "She knows what's coming, and she can't do a damn thing about it."

"Maybe she needs a little reminder to be obedient," another man said with a wicked grin. "Let's make sure she knows exactly what we expect from her this week."

As the men continued to discuss how best to reinforce my submission, I couldn't help but feel my arousal grow despite the terror gnawing at my insides.

"Guys! Why a sex pet? Sex slave sounds better to me!"

These men seemed to have an unquenchable thirst for my suffering. My clitoris seemed to call out to them, and the hunger in their eyes was unmistakable. I had always wanted to be at the mercy of a group of men, letting their most basic barbarian instincts lose, and my wildest fantasies had finally come true as I lay at the mercy of these old men, experiencing a terror unlike any other and yet strangely aroused by the prospect of being brutalized.

"Right! We trained her as a sex pet, but now you gotta train her as a sex slave, Harvey!"

"Alright then," Harvey finally declared, holding the dreaded black binder paper clip in his hand. "Let's make a sex slave out of her."

My body tensed as he approached, the cold metal of the clip glinting menacingly. The other men watched with eager anticipation, their faces twisted with cruel delight.

"Remember, sweetheart," a man taunted, his voice dripping with sadistic glee, "this is what happens when you don't behave like an obedient sex slave."

My eyes widened in terror, and I tried to scream through the gag, but all that emerged were pitiful whimpers. What's the point of a safe word if you are gagged? The men's laughter filled the room as they reveled in my helplessness, their twisted amusement only fueling my own dark desires.

"Ah, there it is," one man murmured, his eyes locked on my fear-stricken face. "That look of desperation, of pure submission... it's intoxicating. She's so fuckin' beautiful!"

"Damn right, she is," another agreed, his voice thick with lust. "I can't wait to see her break down completely under our control. Never had a sex slave before. And certainly not a babe like her!"

I struggled against the iron grip of two men who had spontaneously taken hold of my thighs to push them apart, my body writhing in a futile attempt to escape their grasp. Their laughter rang in my ears as they reveled in my distress, my humiliation fueling their evil desires.

"Look at her squirm," one man chuckled, his eyes glinting with sadistic glee. "She's not some damsel in distress—she's the damsel we're going to put in distress."

"Damn right," another agreed, licking his lips as he stared at my exposed, vulnerable form. "We'll teach this little slut what a clit is for. Fuck clits!"

Harvey stood in front of me with the binder clip in hand, his expression cold and merciless. He asked the men to release their hold on my thighs, and they stepped back to their comfortable chairs. I immediately closed my legs, but Harvey shot me a stern look that made it clear any resistance would only make things worse.

"Listen up, baby girl," he growled, holding the binder clip menacingly before my face. "I'm only going to put this on your clit for one minute, just to make sure you understand the consequences if you disobey us."

"Or if she sucks our cocks like shit," one man chimed in, his words sending a shiver down my spine.

"Or if her pussy ain't tight enough for our liking," added another, eliciting approving nods from the others.

It seemed to me they were more excited by finding any reason to torture my clit than by fucking me.

Tears welled up in my eyes as the weight of my situation bore down on me. My heart pounded in my chest, my body trembling in fear. Yet, beneath the terror, there was an undeniable euphoria—a perverse excitement at being so utterly at the mercy of these men.

"Please," I whimpered, though my muffled plea went unnoticed due to the ball gag filling my mouth. The men laughed at my feeble attempt to beg for mercy, their amusement only serving to further degrade me.

"Look at her, trying to speak with that dildo gag in her mouth," one man taunted. "Your mouth is only for sucking, babe!"

"Enough," Harvey snapped. Fixing his gaze on me, he repeated his demand. "One minute, Delisha. And if you don't cooperate, it'll only be worse for you."

His words echoed in my mind as I reluctantly nodded. Yet, I simply couldn't open my legs as if they refused to obey me. The room fell silent, anticipation hanging heavy in the air as they watched, waiting for the moment when my body would be racked with agony once more.

"Two minutes, Delisha," Harvey announced, his voice dripping with authority. My heart raced as I hesitated, my legs trembling in fear. With a shaky breath, I reluctantly opened them halfway.

"Ha! Look at her, just like watching a football game and waiting for the next touchdown," one man called out, earning chuckles from the others.

"More like a wrestling match where we're all rooting for the bad guy," another chimed in, licking his lips as he stared hungrily at my exposed body.

"Three minutes, Delisha," Harvey announced, his eyes never leaving mine. Desperate to avoid further suffering, I finally forced my legs wide open, tears streaming down my cheeks.

"Good girl," Harvey praised, a sadistic grin spreading across his face. The men around me hooted and hollered, eager to see what would happen next.

"Alright, Delisha, since you've been so compliant, I'm going to remove your handcuffs," Harvey declared, unlocking the cold metal cuffs from my wrists. "Now spread those pretty pussy lips for us and push your hood aside."

My hands trembled as they moved toward my scared pussy, but the humiliation and fear were too much for me to bear. Instead of obeying, I covered my private female parts, sobbing uncontrollably.

"Four minutes it is then," Harvey announced without any hint of sympathy. The men erupted into laughter and crude comments, reveling in my torment. "Make it ten already!"

"Look at her trying to protect that little clit of hers," one teased.

"Enough!" Harvey snapped, silencing the room. "Open up, or it'll be even worse."

Taking a deep, shuddering breath, I mustered the courage to reveal my most sensitive part to my torturer. My hands quivered as I spread my outer labia, fear coursing through me like an electric shock. I thrust my hood back, leaving my clit exposed and vulnerable to Harvey's malicious intent. Every beat of my heart felt like a sledgehammer pounding in my chest as I stared into Harvey's eyes, pleading for mercy that I knew would never come.

"Look at her," Theo chuckled, "so desperate for it."

"Ball gag off," Harvey decided, reaching down and unfastening the strap from around my head. The dildo slipped out of my mouth, and I gasped for air. "Now tell me you want it."

"Please, no!" I cried, tears streaming down my face. "I don't want it!"

"Ha! She doesn't want it, boys," Edgar taunted. "But we all know she needs it."

"Five minutes then," Harvey announced, smirking at my anguish. The men erupted into cheers and crude laughter, reveling in my torment.

"Please, please, no!" I begged, sobbing uncontrollably. But my pleas only seemed to fuel their sadistic desires.

"Spread wider, slut," Francis jeered. "Show us that pretty little clit of yours."

"Come on, Harvey, make her scream," Wilfred urged, his eyes gleaming with malicious delight.

"Alright, Delisha," Harvey said, his voice cold and detached. "Do you understand your role as our sex slave?"

I nodded through my tears, barely able to get the words out. "Yes, I understand."

"Say it," he demanded, gripping the binder paper clip menacingly. "Tell us all how much you deserve this punishment."

"I... I deserve this punishment," I stammered, hating myself for giving in to their twisted demands.

"Why?" Harvey asked, his grip on the clip tightening.

"Because I am a cock tease. And a dumb blonde."

"Right! And when will we put this binder clip on your clit?"

"Whenever any of you are not pleased with me," I repeated, choking on the words and my hands shaking as I kept holding my outer lips apart to expose my clit, "you should punish my clit with it."

"Good girl," he sneered, bringing the clip closer. My body trembled as I braced for the agony to come.

"Please, Harvey," I whimpered one last desperate plea.

"Too late for begging now, sweetheart," he replied, his voice devoid of sympathy.

With a swift motion, he snapped the binder paper clip onto my swollen clit, and an indescribable pain shot through me. As I writhed and sobbed, the men jeered and laughed, reveling in my excruciating torment.

The pain that surged through me as Harvey snapped the tight metal binder paper clip onto my exposed clit was unbearable. My legs gave out, and I crumpled to the porch floor like a broken doll. Through tear-filled eyes, I glimpsed one of the old men smirking at my plight.

"Look at her," he chuckled darkly. "Like a deflated inflated doll."

"Damn! Look at her go!" Stanley cheered, excitement in his voice. "I've never seen anything more beautiful! Fuckin' erotic!"

"Music to my ears," David added, grinning wickedly as my cries filled the air.

"Five minutes of pure bliss," Cliff mused, leaning back in his chair and watching me twist and shake with dark satisfaction.

Desperate to end the torment, I brought my trembling hands to my throbbing clit and managed to remove the clip. But my relief was short-lived as the men's expressions turned angry.

"Didn't give you permission to take it off, slut," Harvey growled, his face contorted with rage. "Now it'll be six minutes. Reset."

I sobbed uncontrollably as I once again forced my legs apart and pushed my outer lips aside, exposing my tender clit to the cruel clip. The anticipation made me shake even more violently as Harvey slowly inched the clip toward my most sensitive spot.

"Say it, bitch," he commanded, his voice dripping with malice. "Beg me to put it on."

"Please, Harvey," I whimpered, tears streaming down my cheeks. "Please put it on."

"Tell me again why you want it," he taunted, pausing with the clip hovering just above my clit.

"Please, I want it," I choked on my own words. "I'm a cock tease."

"Tell me more, babe," he demanded, moving the clip ever so slightly closer.

"Please, please," I stammered, desperate for this twisted game to end, "put it on my clit. I deserve to be punished."

"Tell... me... more, slave girl."

"Please, Harvey!" I cried out, barely able to speak through my sobs. "You guys can punish my clit anytime you are not pleased with me."

"Anytime? Like in... Anytime?"

"Yes," I could barely articulate, my hands shaking so much that I could hardly hold my pussy lips apart to expose my clit to my torturer and to the spectators waiting to see the young blonde suffer.

"Who can do it?"

"Any of you!" I added, choking on my words more than ever. "Any of you, any time, you can beat my clit."

Satisfied by my broken pleas, Harvey finally snapped the clip back onto my pulsating clit. The pain was even more intense than before, and I writhed on the rough porch floor, my body convulsing with every heartbeat. The men watched with dark satisfaction as I suffered for their twisted amusement.

Every second seemed more like a minute, and they wanted the babe to suffer for 360 seconds. I couldn't help but squirm as my body convulsed on the porch, first on my back like a piece of bacon in a hot pan, then on my side, and then returning to my back again. With every heartbeat, the pain radiated throughout my entire body, leaving me breathless and desperate for relief.

The thought of using my safe word crossed my mind, but something within me resisted. I wanted to prove that I could endure this torment for these men.

Besides, I knew I would share this sexual experience with you guys, and knowing your cocks would also get hard motivated me even more.

"Look at her go," one of them chuckled as they watched me writhe in agony. "It's about damn time a fuckin' clit got what it deserves."

"Damn right," another agreed, his voice dripping with disdain. "I've had to please my wife's clit for years. It's pathetic how much attention those little things demand."

"Isn't it amazing watching such a beautiful girl suffer like this?" Theo asked, a wicked grin spreading across his face. "I never thought we would have such an erotic show when I paid my deposit for this trip."

"Her pussy must be feeling so sorry for itself right now," David added, smirking at my humiliation. "I bet she'll think twice before being a cock tease again."

"Remember all those times our wives forced us to go down on them?" Fred chimed in, his words filled with bitterness. "Well, there it is, sweetheart! We'll go down on you all week, babe... with a binder paper clip!"

"Think about it, boys," Albert said, rubbing his hands together. "Once we break her, we can use her clit however we want. I want to see her beg for the binder clip again."

"Talk about sweet revenge," Edgar muttered, a cruel smile playing on his lips. "Fuck you, clit!"

I listened to their cruel laughter and taunting words, feeling my humiliation deepen with each passing moment. I couldn't help but think of my parents and how they encouraged me to be happy in my wild pursuits. And even as I writhed in pain, a part of me took pride in enduring this brutal treatment for the entertainment of the men surrounding me. It was a twisted, perverse sense of accomplishment that kept me from using my safe word. I wanted my mom and dad to be proud of me.

"Look at her," Harvey said, pointing at my trembling form. "She's barely hanging on, but she's still not using her safe word. She must really want to please us."

"Or she's just a glutton for punishment," Theo suggested with a wicked grin. "Either way, we win."

The pain didn't get better. In fact, it intensified, but so did my determination. I could feel the men's eyes on me, feasting upon my agony, and I knew that I would endure this torment for them.

In a world where these old men felt powerless, I would give them the control they craved, even if it meant suffering through this unbearable pain.

I've always wanted to be the cure for emasculation.

My body never stopped trembling on the porch, convulsing with each agonizing throb of pain from the binder clip crushing my clit. Hot tears streamed down my cheeks as I struggled to stay strong, to resist the temptation to use my safe word or my hands to end this torment.

"See how she tries to remove it?" Harvey taunted, watching my hands hover over the clip but never quite reach it. "But she knows better, don't you, babe? If you remove it, we reset the clock and make it ten minutes."

"Fuck! I hope she takes it off!" a laughing voice said.

"Ya! That'd be cool," Stanley agreed, a sinister grin spreading across his face. "She thought she was so high and mighty when she tortured our cocks in our pants with her half-naked body at Miami airport yesterday. Now look at her, writhing in pain like a worm on a hook."

"About time one of those stuck-up blonde bitches got put in her place," Cliff added, his eyes gleaming with malicious delight. "Look who's laughing now, sweetheart! We have control over your body, we decide when and how you feel pleasure or pain."

"Pain!" another man corrected. "Pain only. No pleasure for her."

"She's on an island, naked, with no passport. She's an animal!"

My heart pounded in my chest, and I could feel their leering gazes upon my naked, helpless form. It was true; they had complete power over me, and there was nothing I could do about it. But even as the pain threatened to consume me, I felt a perverse satisfaction in the thought that I was giving these men what they craved, that I was submitting to their darkest desires and making them feel like real men.

"Bet she never imagined she'd end up like this when she decided to organize this sex & scuba trip," Wilfred sneered, folding his arms across his chest. "Squirming in agony while we watch and laugh. Turns out she's even more beautiful like that."

"Let's see her try to act all high and mighty now," Francis chuckled darkly. "Hard to look down on someone when you're on your back, crying and begging for mercy."

"Maybe she'll think twice before teasing us again," Victor taunted. "Not that she'll have much time to worry about that—after all, she'll get a whole week of hard fun."

As they continued to mock and jeer at my pain, I gritted my teeth and fought back the urge to scream out my safe word even though I ended up dizzy, and nausea invaded my throat.

"Gosh! Is she gonna vomit the sperm we gave her so generously?" a man asked to the general laughter.

The humiliation was unbearable, but I was determined to prove to them—and to myself, my parents, and my best friend—that I could endure this torment, that I was strong enough to withstand their cruelty.

"Get used to it, sweetheart. This is just the first day of our vacation... Remember scuba diving? Nah! Not for you! *This* is for you."

As they continued to mock me, I forced myself to think about how proud I'd be to tell my parents about my latest sexual exploit. How impressed they'd surely be that I'd endured such torment at the hands of a group of old men. It was a twisted thought, but it gave me just enough strength to keep going.

"Look at her! That sure is a lot of crying," Albert sneered. "Thought she could handle it, did she? Bet she's never been put in her place like this before."

Through my tear-blurred vision, I saw them all sitting comfortably around me, enjoying the show I was providing, watching me suffer with wicked grins on their faces. Their vulgar remarks and cruel laughter fueled my resolve to endure the terrors, to prove that I could withstand whatever they had in store for me.

"Think she'll make it through the week?" Charles asked, smirking at my writhing form.

"Who knows?" Cliff shrugged, his eyes gleaming with malicious anticipation. "But I'm sure as hell looking forward to finding out."

As the seconds ticked slowly by and the pain continued to pulse through my body, I clung to the thought of how proud I'd be when I'd tell my parents about this experience. How impressed they'd be at my resilience, my strength, and my unwavering determination to honor old men and worship old cocks. My Mom and Dad always encouraged me to push my sexual limits and experiment to find new sensations.

"Your parents will be so proud," I whispered to myself, tears streaming down my face as I forced myself to bear the agony. "You can do this. You can do this."

And with each second that passed, my resolve grew stronger, and the fire within me burned hotter.

12

A Painful Barefoot Walk of Shame on Gravel

My body ached from the relentless torture inflicted upon my tender clit by those 14 barbarian men. Their eagerness to see me suffer was evident in their lust-filled eyes, feasting on my pain and torment as I twisted and convulsed before them. The memory of the unforgiving binder paper clip still haunted me, and I knew they eagerly anticipated my disobedience to give them an excuse for another erotic show. Even my tears, which streamed down my cheeks while they abused my helpless body, seemed to fuel their depraved desires.

There I was now, walking with the 14 old men towards the restaurant for lunch, reduced to a docile, submissive sex slave. They had won. They owned me. And my heart raced with fear and anticipation while my mind replayed the brutal treatment I had endured.

"Look at her tits bounce," one man growled, his eyes locked onto my heaving chest. "Makes me wanna grab 'em and twist those pretty pink nipples."

"Can't wait till we get to the restaurant," another chimed in, his voice thick with lust, "Imagine all those other guys staring at her, wishing they could have a piece of her sweet ass."

My humiliation only intensified with every crude comment they made, but I didn't dare object. I knew what would happen if I did: more excruciating pain, more savage treatment, more tears.

As we continued along the trail under the palm trees, I tried to focus on anything other than their lewd remarks. But every tug on my leash, every cruel laugh, and every lascivious gaze served as a constant reminder that I was now their property – a submissive, defeated female body with only one purpose: pleasing these men, either visually or physically, lovingly, tenderly, erotically, or violently as they wished.

My bare feet ached as they hit the ground. The handcuffs bit into my wrists, held tightly behind my back. A shiny butt plug nestled inside me, reminding me of its presence with every step. My neck was encircled by a choker collar, and a five-inch dildo ball gag filled my mouth, pushing against my throat and making speech impossible. My captors had made it clear that for the entire week, my mouth would be servicing them, whether wrapped around the rubber phallus or their own eager cocks.

"Can't believe we have this sexy little babe all to ourselves for a whole week," another chimed in as they all exchanged knowing looks. "Her body is a fucking playground. Head to toe!"

"Those ankle restraints are a nice touch," a man added, eyeing the cuffs that adorned my slender ankles. "Perfect for tying her legs together or chaining her up when we want her helpless."

The rude comments continued as we walked, each man taking turns to express his perverse interest in my body and what they planned to do with it. I focused on putting one foot in front of the other, trying to ignore the pain and humiliation that seemed to be my constant companions since we arrived at the dive resort less than 24 hours ago.

"Hey, boys," one of the men called out, drawing everyone's attention. "Check this out." He reached forward and gave the leash a sharp tug, causing the collar to constrict around my neck. I gasped and stumbled, struggling to breathe as he held the tension. Eventually, he relented, releasing the pressure just enough for me to draw in a ragged breath.

"Did you see her face?" he laughed, turning to the others. "She is so fuckin' beautiful like that."

"Let me have a go," another demanded, reaching for the leash and repeating the cruel action. This continued on as they took turns choking me with the collar, each man eager to exert his dominance over my vulnerable form and admire how attractive I was when choking.

My body trembled with pain and exhaustion, but I knew there would be no mercy from these sadistic men. They owned me now, body and soul, and I was nothing more than an object for them to use and abuse as they saw fit. And I fuckin' loved it!

"Keep walking, sweetheart," one of them barked, giving the leash another harsh tug. "We wouldn't want you to disappoint us by passing out before we get there."

Stumbling along the palm tree-lined trail, my body ached from the abuse it had already endured. The 14 men surrounding me reveled in their ownership of my once-proud form, reduced to a submissive, defeated naked plaything.

"Look at that tight ass," one man leered, slapping my exposed buttocks.

"Her tits are perfect, too," another chimed in, reaching forward to roughly grope my breasts. "I bet she loves having them slapped and bitten."

I felt a bitter satisfaction coursing through me as I watched the group of men around me, their eyes glistening with vicious pleasure. They had taken my request for rough treatment and twisted it into something beyond my wildest imagination. My body was wracked with pain and pleasure, but I refused to let my expression betray me. This was what I craved, what I lived for – to be used and abused by those who understood my needs. And these men understood them more than any others ever had before. I couldn't help but wonder just how far they would go or if there would even be anything left of me when they were done. And yet, despite the fear that gnawed at my insides, I knew I wouldn't stop them. Not now, not ever.

"Maybe we should just tie her up and let everyone at the resort have a go," someone suggested, chuckling darkly. "Imagine the look on their faces when they see this perfect little fucktoy, all tied up and ready for use."

"Fuck yeah," another man growled, reaching out to grope my ass again. "This is going to be the best dive trip of our lives."

The harsh sun beat down on me as I kept walking barefoot alongside the 14 old men, their eyes fixated on my naked body. My feet pressed against the rough gravel and occasional rocks beneath them, each step sending a jolt of pain through my legs. I couldn't help but slow down, the ache in my feet causing my buttocks to tighten with every careful step.

"Look at how her ass clenches when she steps on rocks," one man observed, licking his lips. "It is so beautiful!"

"Damn right," another chimed in, grinning wickedly. "It's so fucking hot watching her struggle like that, knowing we own every inch of that tight little body."

"Her ass cheeks are like two perfect mounds of flesh, clenching and releasing with each painful step," a third man added, his eyes locked onto my behind. "Makes me want to shove my cock between those cheeks right now."

As I continued walking, my feet aching more and more, the men seemed to grow increasingly excited by the sight of my contracting buttocks. The pain in my feet was excruciating, but I couldn't deny that some twisted part of me enjoyed this perverse attention to my buttocks.

"Hey boys, let's make sure she keeps stepping on those rocks," one man suggested. "We don't want to miss out on this tasty view."

“Well, take that off,” another one said as he abruptly pulled the butt plug out of my butthole. “See? Butthole clenches too!”

"God, I can't wait to fuck that ass later," someone else muttered, clearly aroused by my pain and vulnerability. "You know, guys, we need to find a way for her to be in pain while we fuck her ass. Imagine the cock massage!"

I tried to step onto the grass at the side of the trail, hoping to find some relief for my aching feet. The men surrounding me didn't seem to appreciate that, however.

"Get back on the rocks, babe," one of them growled, yanking my leash, so I stumbled back onto the painful gravel. "We want to see that tight ass of yours clench with every step."

"Please," I tried to mumble through the ball gag, feeling the sting of tears in my eyes as the rocks bit into my tender soles.

"You deserve it, fucking blonde cock tease," another man sneered, his grip tightening around my leash.

"Damn! Watching you suffer is fucking hot," another added, reaching out to slap my ass, making me wince. "Never seen anything more erotic in my life."

The thought of being utterly at their mercy, completely helpless and vulnerable, continued to stir something dark and twisted within me. A strange cocktail of fear and lust left me reeling, unsure of what to expect from the rest of the week.

I continued to stumble forward slowly on the gravel, my feet aching from the sharp rocks that dug into my bare feet. The men around me watched with keen interest, their eyes glued to my nude, tortured ass as it tightened and relaxed with each agonizing step.

"Damn, look at those cheeks clench," one of the men commented, his voice dripping with lewd desire. "I want to feel that tightness around my cock. You are right, man! She needs to be in pain when we pound her ass!"

One by one, the 14 men took turns standing behind me, reaching out to grip my asscheeks firmly in their hands as I continued walking on the rocky terrain. Each time I stepped onto a particularly sharp rock, I couldn't help but yelp, which only seemed to arouse them further.

"Fuck, that feels amazing," one man groaned, squeezing my ass as I winced in pain. "She's like a living sex toy, perfectly responsive to our touch."

"Damn you, guys," another chimed in, his fingers digging into my flesh as if trying to claim ownership. "You're right! Imagine how good it would feel to fuck her while she's squirming in pain like this."

Their crude comments and rough handling only served to emphasize the cruel reality of my situation – I was nothing more than an object to them, a plaything to be used and abused for their erotic pleasure. And for them, a young, sexy babe in tears was erotic. It wasn't the first time I had encountered such a phenomenon. Many men seem to be turned out by a chick in tears – a blonde one, anyway.

I remember thinking at that moment about the walk of shame Cersei Lannister had to do in the nude through the streets of King's Landing in Game of Thrones. I was tougher than her! She didn't have gravel under her feet.

"Keep walking, baby girl," one of them growled as they continued to take turns gripping my ass, relishing the sensation of my muscles contracting beneath their touch. "You're here to amuse us, remember? And so far, so good."

A shudder ran through me as I struggled to hold back tears, my body aching from both the physical pain and the fear of future pain they kept promising. But deep down, the darkness within me craved their rough manhandling of my small body. I had to admit I wanted more.

How much pain could I endure before using my safe word? 'Never' is what I wanted to prove.

13

My Young Nude Female Body Put On Display For 31 Old Men To Touch

As I stood there, the cool breeze brushing against my exposed flesh, I felt a perverse sense of satisfaction. The 14 old men had led me into the restaurant, my young female body nude from head to toe, tethered by a collar and leash. My feet and clitoris throbbed in pain from the lessons the old men had given me to break me and make me accept to be their sex slave for the week. They own me now. And the exhibitionist in me reveled in the attention. All around the room, the conversation had ceased as 17 other divers stared, their eyes filled with lust and hunger.

"Damn, look at this blonde bombshell," one of the strangers muttered, his gaze locked onto my heaving breasts.

"Fuck yeah," another chimed in, leering at my fully waxed pussy.

My mind swam with their words, my submissive nature awakening. Instead of feeling ashamed or humiliated, I felt an intoxicating mix of fear and arousal. This was what I craved—to be objectified, desired, consumed by bestial old men, and so few men were willing to indulge me. This was a week in paradise for me.

The 14 men who owned me for the week gathered around a few tables, discussing their plans for their fuck doll. Unable to eat anything but sperm all week, I listened to their crude whispers and suggestions.

"Let's have her climb on the table, spread her legs wide, and make a show of it," one suggested, his voice raspy with hunger.

"Damn right," another agreed, rubbing his hands together. "We should let everyone see what a gorgeous fucktoy we've got here."

Others argued that I should be made to crawl beneath the tables, servicing their cocks while they ate.

Finally, they decided to place me atop a table.

As some of the 14 men who owned me began arranging a table for me, the other 17 strangers couldn't help but comment on my body—my firm boobs, my smooth-waxed pussy, my toned body shining with sweat.

"Fuck, look at those tits," one man said, his breath heavy with lust.

"Her ass looks so inviting, too," another added, his eyes locked on my bare buttocks. "Can you imagine slapping those cheeks as you ram your cock deep inside her?"

"Christ, she's like fucking Aphrodite," a third whispered, unable to tear his gaze away from my exposed slit. "I bet she tastes like heaven."

Soon, I found myself being guided onto a table by the rough hands owning my body. One of them commanded, "Get on your knees, babe, but spread 'em wide." I complied, feeling the cold surface of the table beneath me as I positioned myself to fully expose my bald, young pussy to the leering gazes of 31 old men.

"Arch your back, girl," another man ordered, his eyes fixed on my perky breasts. I did as I was told, pushing my chest out, accentuating my firm tits while the men around me licked their lips in anticipation.

"Now, look down and don't make eye contact with any of us unless we tell you to," Harvey instructed, his voice stern. I nodded and lowered my gaze, focusing on the floor as if it held all the answers to life's mysteries.

As I knelt there, exposed and vulnerable, I could hear the other 17 men, some of whom were discovering my nude body for the first time. Their voices carried excitement and arousal that sent shivers down my spine.

"Jesus Christ, would you look at that babe?" one man exclaimed, his voice filled with awe. "She's like a fucking wet dream come true."

"Those tits are just... perfect," another commented, his words laced with lust. "Can you imagine seeing them bouncing while you fuck her?"

"Her tiny pussy looks so tight and... Gosh, erotic," a third chimed in, his longing obvious.

Their words only fueled my desire to be objectified and used by these men. I reveled in their admiration, knowing that my nude body was the center of attention and the focus of their raw desires. My body. Me.

Since my teenage years, I've always enjoyed being nude, especially around old men. And even though it is politically incorrect, I've always been thrilled when objectified. I don't know why it is considered bad since it actually puts me in control. They all want me. Me!

AS THE 14 men who owned me and the 17 other scuba divers devoured their lunch, my body remained on display like a delectable dessert. I had accepted my defeat, knowing that I was now nothing more than a sex pet—correction, a sex slave—to be objectified for their pleasure. My mind didn't even entertain the idea of protest; I was a submissive toy for them to use and admire.

"Damn," one of the 17 men muttered between bites, his gaze fixated on my exposed pussy. "I've never seen anything so fucking perfect."

"Can you imagine what it feels like to be inside her?" another chimed in, licking his lips as he stared at my naked form. Their crude words only fueled my desire to serve as their ultimate sex object.

After everyone had finished eating, they naturally gravitated toward me, encircling the table like a pack of hungry wolves. The air buzzed with curiosity and arousal as the 17 other male scuba divers questioned my owners about how this all came to be.

"Seriously, how did you guys arrange this?" one of the 17 asked. "We were told there'd be a college girl nude all week for some school project, but we never thought she'd be this stunning. She's like a goddamn Playboy Playmate!"

"Right place, right time," Harvey replied smugly, stroking my hair possessively. "Seriously, Delisha is actually the one who organized the trip. She recruited us!"

I felt a thrill run through me at his words, knowing that my behavior was shocking to so many of them. So few people understand—and even fewer accept—my sexual needs.

"Her body is just... incredible," a man from the 17 commented, his eyes roving over me hungrily. "I can't believe how firm and perky her tits are. And that ass... God, I'd love to spank it."

"Everything about her is perfect," another agreed, his gaze lingering on my bald pussy. "How is she in the sack? I bet she's wild."

Their lewd comments continued as they inspected every inch of me, admiring and lusting after my body as if I were a priceless work of art. And in a way, I was—an erotic masterpiece crafted to fulfill their deepest, darkest desires.

Through it all, I kept my gaze lowered, obediently following Harvey's instructions never to look any man in the eyes unless ordered to. My submission only added to their excitement.

My body ached from being immobile for so long as an erotic centerpiece, but I didn't dare move or complain. I'd been beaten into submission, and my purpose now was to provide amusement for these old men. They devoured me with their eyes during lunch, and I reveled in the feeling of being objectified.

Conversations between the 17 other scuba divers grew more animated as they discussed what they'd witnessed so far. Those who had seen me being spit-roasted earlier on the dive boat eagerly shared details with those who hadn't.

"Man, you should've seen her," one of them said, his voice filled with excitement. "She was like a wild animal, taking both cocks without any hesitation. Her mouth wrapped around one while the other pounded her tight pussy. It was hot."

"Fuck, I wish I'd seen that," another chimed in, clearly aroused by the image.

"Her tiny pussy looked so fucking good stretched around a cock," a third added, licking his lips. "And the sounds she made... God, it was like music to my ears."

As they described me in such crude terms, a part of me felt degraded, but another part—the darker, twisted side—craved their approval.

Among the 17 men who were new to the experience, discussions centered around their surprise at discovering the nudity experiment included sex and how utterly entranced they were by my model-like body. They said it, not me!

"Her tits are just perfect," one man commented, staring openly at my chest. "They're so firm and perky, like they're defying gravity."

"Her ass is a work of art, too," another agreed, his hand making a lewd-grabbing motion in the air.

"Never seen a bald pussy like that before," a third man said, his gaze fixated on my exposed sex. "It's like she was made for fucking."

I was so thrilled by these last words. For a long time now, I've been thinking that my body was specifically designed to be a fuck doll, and finding men who agreed with me was always a delight.

"Look, boys," Harvey, one of the 14 men who owned me for the week, announced to the other scuba divers, "feel free to touch her anywhere you want. We own her body and soul, but we're more than happy to share her skin."

As if on cue, the 17 other men's hands reached out to explore my flesh. I felt a shiver of anticipation and anxiety running through me, unsure of what to expect.

"Her ass is so smooth," a man chanted, caressing my buttocks with a lewd grin on his face before adding a slap with a sting that only added to my intoxicating mix of pain and pleasure.

"Bet this tight pussy feels amazing around a cock," a third man observed, his fingers daring to graze over my sensitive folds. I bit my lip, struggling not to react to their rude remarks and how casually they were touching my pussy.

"Man, just look at her nipples," another diver said, pinching and twisting them as I tried to stifle a moan. "I'd love to suck on those."

The men continued to grope and fondle every inch of my body, their vulgarity growing by the minute. Their hands roamed my skin, leaving behind marks as they reveled in my humiliation and submission.

"Her belly button looks so cute with that piercing," one old man noted, poking his finger into my navel, causing me to flinch.

"And her thighs... Man! So toned," another admired, squeezing them with a firm grip. "Guys! Imagine these thighs wrapped around your waist."

"Even her feet are sexy," a third diver mused, lifting one of my legs to inspect my delicate toes and arches.

"Come on, boys, don't be shy!" one of the older men who claimed ownership over me shouted to the others who had not touched me yet. "We're all friends here, and we've got a beautiful piece of meat to share."

"Exactly," another chimed in, his eyes locked onto my exposed pussy.

The other men, their eyes filled with lustful hunger, moved in, their hands reaching out to finally explore every inch of my body.

As I felt rough fingers dig into my tender flesh, I felt a perverse ecstasy at being treated like a mere object. Each touch sent shivers down my spine as I imagined what dirty thoughts they had.

As they continued to inspect me, probing my most intimate areas as if they were shopping for a fuck doll, I could only focus on their crude words and actions. Each comment and touch fueled my desire to be used and degraded, knowing that I existed solely for their carnal pleasure.

Harvey's order had made me immobile, unable to resist or react as the hands of strangers continued to run over my exposed flesh. And my boobs were popular!

"Her stomach is so flat," one man remarked, running his hand along the curve of my waist and down to my hips. "Perfect for holding onto while you pound her from behind."

"Absolutely," a third agreed, moving his attention to my ass. He slapped it hard, making me gasp as the sting vibrated through my sensitive skin. "And this ass... it's like it was made for spanking."

31 men around me laughed, exchanging crude comments about what they'd do to me as they took turns exploring every inch of my body. Some played with my long blonde hair, winding it around their fingers and tugging at it, while others traced the contours of my nose and cheeks. My feet weren't spared either, as they caressed and squeezed them, admiring their delicate shape.

Since I started exploring my sexuality as a teenager, I have fantasized about moments like this, craving old men to objectify me completely, giving no thought to my humanity. I had the chance to experience it a few times, but the atmosphere on this tropical island was making it more satisfying.

At prior sex parties, I often had to insist and sometimes even beg the men to use me as their plaything unless my friend Madison was there to coach them—but not here. Here, I was thoroughly objectified, a source of amusement meant only for their pleasure. They were not afraid to be rough and even violent. The intensity of the situation sent my senses reeling, and I couldn't help but crave more and more depraved exploration in the coming days; little did I know that the rest of the day would, in itself, be a challenge.

14

The 14 Men Owning Me Already Planned Another Dive Trip For 54 Divers With My Body On The Menu

My nude young female body, put on display on the table like a succulent feast for hungry eyes, gleamed in the early afternoon light. The group of 14 men who owned me and the additional 17 who had just joined stared with ravenous desire. I felt their hands exploring every inch of my naked flesh, rough fingers pinching and grabbing, even daring to casually delve into my wet pussy.

"Hey, what's this 'spermivore' written on her toenails?" one of the 17 men asked, his fingers caressing my bare feet.

"Means she only eats sperm, semen," Theo explained with a smirk. "She's addicted to it."

"Can't blame the girl," another man from the group of 17 said as he gazed at my naked body. "If all women followed that diet, they might look as fucking irresistible as this slut here."

The thought of being responsible for setting a trend among young women both amused and excited me.

"Damn, that's hot," one of the newcomers chimed in. "I wouldn't mind donating some sperm to her cause."

"Same here," agreed another, his eyes roaming over my exposed flesh.

A heated discussion ensued among the men about whether or not they should share me, their living fuck doll. The 14 members of my group explained that they had undergone health checks before embarking on this adventure to ensure they could fuck me whenever they pleased.

After much debate, the group of 14 took a vote and decided to share me with the other 17 men, but with certain conditions: no blowjobs for sperm donations, and condoms had to be used for my ass and pussy.

My heart raced as I listened to old men discussing what to do with my young body, never once asking for my opinion or consent, although, of course, they knew I had a safe word if I really wanted to object. Well, I had a dildo gag and couldn't speak, but... Don't confuse me with facts!

In any case, it was thrilling to be owned by these men, who saw me as nothing more than an erotic plaything to share.

"Alright, then," Harvey declared, satisfied with their decision. "You can use her body; just follow our rules."

I reveled in the sensation of being at the mercy of so many men, my body aching with anticipation for the debauchery that was sure to follow.

The erotic thrill of the situation intensified as some of the 17 newcomers eagerly expressed their desire to be on the next trip with me, craving my blowjobs and the chance to further use my body for their pleasure. The general manager, grasping an opportunity to save his struggling dive resort, started jotting down the names of the scuba divers who were willing to book a trip if I was part of the tempting package.

"Count us all in," one of the men from the group of 17 interjected, a wicked grin etched on his face. "If she's on the menu for the next dive trip, we want in too."

"Alright," the general manager agreed, rubbing his hands together with excitement. "There's room for 54 divers at the resort. With Delisha being the main attraction, I'm sure we can sell it out.

Leave it to me; I'll figure out a week when you can have all the cabins and get back to you."

I was awestruck at how much value and desirability these men placed on my body. The thought of having 54 men manhandling me in a tropical paradise for a week gave me shivers, especially if they were as sadistic as the 14 I was currently with. But deep down, the idea excited me. My nipples hardened at the mere thought of being used and abused by so many men. Suddenly, this week was just a dry run, and I fuckin' loved it!

"Listen, guys," Harvey said, addressing the 17 newcomers. "Feel free to pull on her leash and choke her if she doesn't listen or needs the motivation to be a better sexual pet. She's here to please!"

The explicit, graphic language and the violent undertones in their voices made my pussy throb with anticipation. My body was now owned by 14 old men, sharing it with 17 other old men. I was one lucky gal!

Since my teenage years, I've seen old men's cocks as... god! Collectively, these old penises and balls were my god – one I wanted to worship as often as possible. And I had 31 of them for a week on a tropical island. This was paradise. Thank you, god!

"Remember, gentlemen," Harvey reminded them one last time. "Delisha is our property. Don't hold back; let your primal urges take over. But bring her back to us with no permanent physical marks."

Hearing Harvey say that made me love him! Although he was the most sadistic of the group of 14 old men, he had listened to my only non-negotiable rule. I had asked them to give me a beating unless I used my safe word, and they were doing it while making sure I would not end the week with any permanent physical mark.

I was the luckiest girl on earth.

As I remained on the table, my naked body on display for the ravenous gaze of these 31 men, a sudden realization dawned upon the group of 14. Theo spoke up, his voice dripping with lustful excitement, "Boys, we haven't fucked Delisha's sweet ass yet!"

A murmur of agreement rippled through the room as their eyes hungrily roamed over my exposed flesh. My heart raced at the thought of being so thoroughly used and claimed by these men.

"Remember that list of rules she gave us at Miami airport?" Fred asked, chuckling deviously. "She said if we fed her enough sperm during the week, we'd get to bang her ass all night on the last night."

"Fuck those rules," Harvey snorted, grabbing a handful of my blonde hair and yanking my head back, forcing me to look into his eyes. "We're making our own rules now, aren't we, slut?"

I nodded, unable to speak with the dildo ball gag filling my mouth. The prospect of having my ass violated by 14 hard rods excited me beyond belief, reinforcing these men's control and dominance over me.

"Alright then," Stanley declared, rubbing his hands together eagerly. "Let's fuck her ass right now, to remind her just how little her rules mean to us."

The air grew thick with anticipation. The men's crude words made my pussy clenched in response, craving the rough touch of these bestial men even more.

Internally, I marveled at how easily they dismissed my initial boundaries, replacing them with their own twisted desires. It thrilled me that they were eager to take complete ownership of my body, demonstrating their insatiable hunger for my submission. For me!

"Get ready, babe," Victor said, his voice a low growl. "Your tight little ass is about to know the full extent of our desires. And it's just Day One!"

"Let's show her what it means to be completely at our mercy," Harvey said, his dark eyes locked on mine.

I shuddered, my body quivering with anticipation, knowing that my submission to their will would only fuel their bestial hunger for more sex and violence. And in that moment, I realized just how much I craved their domination.

“Take me, please!” I would have yelled if I didn’t have a dildo ball gag.

15

They Pounded My Ass With My Bare Feet on Gravel for My Butthole to Clench, Giving Them a Cock Massage

Surrounded by 14 old men who owned me, my young girl's nude body shivered with anticipation and fear. They had just decided to take turns fucking my ass. Their predatory gazes roamed over my exposed flesh, hunger for dominance fueling their actions.

I had a hard time wrapping my mind around the fact it had been less than 24 hours since we landed for a week-long scuba & sex vacation. Already, my rules had been thrown in the garbage along with my clothing—even my clothes for the flight back. They had beaten me into submission and taken ownership of my body as if they were expert psychopaths.

"Blondie," Victor growled, like a savage beast about to devour his prey. "You know what's coming next, don't you? We're going to fuck that tight little ass of yours until you can't even remember your own name."

The other men in my group of 14 laughed and jeered, egging him on. I felt their eyes on my bare flesh, scanning every inch of my exposed body. My heart raced with a mix of fear and excitement. These men were barbarians, intent on using me for their pleasure—all week!

"Damn straight," Wilfred chimes in, licking his lips obscenely. "I can't wait to pound that sweet ass of yours, make you scream for mercy."

"Let's do it here," a man with a sinister grin suggested, eager to humiliate me further.

"Alright, baby girl," Harvey said, snapping me back to the harsh reality of my situation. "Time to bend over and take what's coming to you."

Trembling, I complied, positioning myself next to a table in the middle of the dive resort restaurant with my ass presented for their taking. The men circled around me like vultures, ready to feast on my vulnerable body.

As a man's hands gripped my hip, ready to thrust into me, another stopped him. "Wait," he said, a twisted grin on his face. "Remember how her ass clenched when she walked barefoot on that gravel? We'll get a better fuck if she's in pain."

The men exchanged lewd comments, vividly describing the eroticism they had found in seeing my ass tighten with each agonizing step on the rocky ground. They reveled in the idea of inflicting pain upon me, their crude words painting a picture of barbaric lust.

"Can you imagine how that tight convulsing hole would feel around your cock?" one man said, his eyes hungry with anticipation.

"Damn right," another cheered, his voice filled with sadistic excitement.

And just like that, the group of old men, still drooling over my naked body, slowly led me around the resort as they searched for the perfect trail. Their eyes scanned the ground, seeking a path covered with the rocks and gravel that would cause my delicate feet the greatest pain. I could tell they were enjoying themselves, their lustful gazes roaming over my curves and settling on my ass, anticipating the rough treatment it would soon receive.

"Look at this one," Edgar pointed to a particularly rocky stretch, grinning wickedly. "Her feet will be in agony on those stones."

"Perfect!" Theo exclaimed, clapping his hands together. "Now, let's see how good she is at milking cocks with her ass."

Before they took what they wanted, which was to feast on my tight young butt, they first desired some entertainment. I was told to make a practice run along the path, and as an obedient sexual object, I did. It made for quite the sight: a young, sexy, nude blonde girl walking barefoot down the gravel path with thirteen old men in sandals flanking either side of her on the grass. Each step felt like a thousand needles stabbing into the soles of my feet. I winced and whimpered, but the men only laughed and taunted me further, my suffering fueling their arousal.

"Aw, does it hurt, sweetheart?" one of them sneered. "Just wait until we're pounding your tight little ass while you suffer on these rocks."

"Such a pretty sight," another chimed in, "Look at it, guys! Watch her ass tense up from the pain. Can't wait to feel that gripping my cock."

"Imagine her squirming beneath us, begging for mercy," a third man said, licking his lips. "That's how we'll really show her who owns her."

As they continued to laugh and jeer, Wilfred stepped forward with an idea. "You know what would make this even more fun? If our little toy here didn't have a ball gag. Then she could beg us to do all kinds of painful things to her while we fuck her hard."

The other men nodded, exchanging excited glances. "Yeah," Fred agreed, reaching forward to unhook the ball gag from my mouth. "Let's hear her pretty voice begging for more."

With the ball gag removed, I could feel their eyes on me, waiting for me to say something. It was as if they were feeding off my pain and humiliation, and it excited me. As the gravel beneath my feet dug into my tender soles, making me wince, I knew they wanted to hear me beg, to see me broken, and somehow, that realization only served to stoke the fire within me.

I also knew I would share this sexual experience with you guys, and knowing your cocks would get hard motivated me even more.

"Please," I gasped, tears already forming in my eyes as I looked up at them. "It hurts so much, but I want your cocks to feel good, so please... fuck my ass while I'm standing on these rocks. Make me suffer for the greater good."

Their leers grew wider, their eyes darkening with lust. They exchanged glances, discussing how they would take turns using me like some kind of pain slut.

"Alright, bitch," Cliff declared, unbuckling his pants. "Since you're asking so nicely, I'll be the first one to pound that tight little hole of yours."

He dropped his pants, revealing his pulsating erection, and the others cheered him on. My heart raced, both from fear and the anticipation of the pain that awaited me. I couldn't believe I was begging out loud for this, and yet, internally, I was indeed begging for it.

I bent forward at the waist while he stood behind me and thrust forward, forcing his thick cock inside me. I cried out in pain—but also in pleasure. I was giving them the show they craved, even as it hurt like hell. The men encouraged Cliff, urging him to be rougher with me, and he obliged, pounding into my ass relentlessly.

"Does that hurt, you little slut?" Edgar taunted from the grassy, comfortable sidelines. "How does it feel to have your ass savagely fucked while your feet are being shredded by these rocks?"

"More... please give me more," I sobbed, though each word felt like a knife to my soul. They enjoyed my pain, and I craved their satisfaction—no matter the cost. "Is it good for your cock?"

"Damn, fuck! It's amazing," Cliff groaned.

As I stumbled forward on the gravel trail, Cliff's iron grip held me firmly by my hips, his hard cock buried deep in my tight ass. Each brutal thrust of his cock beating my ass forced me to take another step, my tender feet screaming in agony with every sharp stone that dug into my soles. The pain caused my butthole to tighten, intensifying the massage Cliff's cock received as he continued to violate me relentlessly.

"Fuck, Delisha, your tight little ass is milking me so good!" he groaned again, his hands tightening around my waist.

I couldn't wait to tell my best friend, Jane. She always thought I was crazy to walk barefoot on gravel as a teenager back home. At the time, I never thought it was the way to give a cock massage!

My body ached, and tears streamed down my cheeks, but I couldn't deny the perverse satisfaction that bloomed inside me. I wanted to be used, to be their cock-pleasuring device, their pain slut, to satisfy their raw desires. Their old men penises deserved to be worshipped, and I was a devotee. If my pain brought them more delight, then I would gladly suffer for them.

"Harder, please," I whimpered, my voice cracking. "Your cock deserves it."

Cliff obliged, slamming his cock into my abused hole with even more force, making me stagger forward. I felt like a ragdoll being tossed around by these ravenous beasts, and that image only fueled my desire to please them more.

"Look at her go, boys!" Theo shouted from behind us, his eyes glued to my trembling form. "She's really begging for it now!"

"And look at those tits wobbling along! Damn, it's fuckin' erotic!"

The other men hooted their approval, their lustful gazes fixated on my naked body. I could feel the weight of their stares, their hunger for my submission, and it only made me ache for more.

"More... please, more," I gasped, the words spilling out of my mouth like a mantra, my body betraying my mind.

The force of Cliff's thrusts was relentless, and I could feel the strain in my abs as I struggled to keep my body at a 90-degree angle. My hands were still handcuffed behind my back, rendering them completely helpless. The pain in my feet from the gravel underfoot was unbearable, but it fueled my desire for more.

"Pull my hair... please," I begged, my voice breaking with desperation.

Cliff smirked, his grip shifting from my waist to my long blonde hair. He yanked it hard, sending a searing pain through my scalp that momentarily distracted me from the agony in my feet and ass. It also provided a brief respite for my overworked abs, a small mercy amidst the torment.

"Like that, you little whore?" he growled, maintaining his hold on my hair as he continued to pound into me.

"Y-yes," I stammered, the pain at the top, bottom, and middle of my body overwhelming yet somehow intoxicating. "Thank you."

With each powerful thrust, Cliff continued to force me to step forward, grinding my tender soles into the sharp rocks below. The sensation was excruciating, and I couldn't help but cry out. But as the pain intensified, so too did the tightness of my buttocks and the contraction of my butthole around his invading cock.

"Fuck, your ass feels incredible when you're hurting like this," Cliff grunted, his face contorted with pleasure.

The other men watched on, their expressions a mixture of lust and sadistic delight. They reveled in my suffering, their eyes feasting upon the vulnerable spectacle I presented.

"Fuck me!" a voice yelled. "Why am I so aroused by this chick crying her heart out? So beautiful!"

"Keep going, Cliff!" Wilfred shouted. "Make her feel every inch of that gravel!"

"More," I whispered, my voice barely audible amidst the cacophony of cheers and jeers. "Make me hurt more. Make me milk your cock better."

The second man, Wilfred, took his place behind me with a lecherous grin. He grabbed a fistful of my long blonde hair and yanked my head back, forcing me to arch my back, delighting the men who had a thing for my young boobs.

"Ready for another round, sweetheart?" he taunted, his voice dripping with malice.

"Please," I whimpered, the pain in my feet throbbing in sync with my racing heart. "Do it."

Wilfred didn't need any more encouragement. He slammed into my ass, causing me to gasp at the sudden intrusion. With each vicious thrust, he tugged on my hair, wrenching my head back further and forcing me to take agonizing steps on the rocky terrain and making my naked tits wobble to the amusement of the spectators.

"Fuck, that's tight," Wilfred grunted, clearly enjoying the way my butthole clenched around him.

My body was wracked with sobs as I struggled to keep my balance on the gravel. The pain was unbearable, and there were 12 more men after him, yet I couldn't deny the perverse thrill that coursed through me as I realized just how much these men were enjoying my torment and, especially, how good it was for my god—the cocks of these men.

"More," I choked out, tears streaming down my face. "Hurt me more. Get what you need for your cock."

"Music to my ears," Wilfred growled, increasing the force of his thrusts and pulling even harder on my hair.

By the time the third man, David, took his turn, we had reached the end of the gravel path. My legs trembled beneath me, my feet aching from the abuse they'd endured.

"Please," I sobbed, the humiliation burning hot in my chest. "Please, make me walk back over the gravel... I want to keep going... for all of you. All."

"Such a good little slut," David praised before roughly shoving me forward.

"Thank you," I whimpered, tears streaming down my cheeks as we retraced my steps. The sensation of being fucked while walking on the jagged rocks beneath my feet was intense and memorable. But knowing that the other men enjoyed the erotic spectacle was nothing but pure joy. I had waited so long for a group of old men to enjoy and abuse my body without me having to coach them non-stop. I was finally living it.

"Your tears are such a fucking turn-on, babe," one of the men leered, his eyes locked onto my face as he relished in my anguish.

For some reason, my young tits and my tears were the biggest hit with these men since we landed on this paradisiac island. Well, and torturing my clit. Top 3!

My body shook with each vicious thrust from Stanley, the fourth man to take his turn. My ass ached and burned, but I could feel my butthole growing tighter around him with every step, giving him the milking effect they craved—the delight my god deserved.

"Look at her tits bounce!" Edgar exclaimed, eyeing me hungrily as my young breasts danced with every violent movement.

"Such a perfect little fucktoy," Charles added, smirking in delight. "The most erotic thing I've ever seen!"

"Make her wobble those tits more, Stan!" Theo urged, laughing as Stanley yanked on my hair even harder, forcing me to arch my back, thrust my chest forward, and put my young tits on display.

I whimpered, but the lewd comments only fueled my twisted desire for pain and humiliation. These old men were treating me like a disposable object, and I couldn't help but crave more.

"Fuck, you guys are right," Stanley grunted, his grip on my hair tightening. "Watching her body squirm in pain is so fucking hot."

"Keep going," Victor yelled, licking his lips with anticipation. "This little cock tease deserves everything she's getting."

As Stanley finally finished inside me, I barely had a moment to catch my breath before Bernard took his place behind me.

"Ready for another round, whore?" Bernard sneered, gripping my hips tightly as he forced his cock into my abused ass. I bit my lip and steeled myself for what was to come.

"Look at this slut," one of the men watching called out. "With that perfect body, she could have any rich sugar daddy she wanted. Never work a day in her life. Never suffer. But here she is, letting us old fucks use her like a cheap whore. What a fucking babe. I think I'm in love!"

"Damn right," another chimed in, eyeing my body hungrily. "It's impressive how much she craves this shit. I think I'm in love, too!"

"Look at her boobs jiggling!" David exclaimed, clearly enjoying the perverse spectacle. "Never seen more beautiful young girl's tits."

"Her face when she's in pain..." Charles mused, grinning wickedly. "It's just so fucking erotic."

"Beautiful, isn't it?" Edgar agreed, his eyes never leaving my tear-streaked face. "And knowing she wants it makes it even better. Fuck my wife! I wanna marry this babe!"

"More," I choked out, my voice barely audible above the sounds of my own tortured sobbing. "Get a good cock massage, please."

"Hey, guys," Bernard said thoughtfully, stroking his chin. "Imagine how much tighter her ass would squeeze our cocks if we clamped that juicy clit of hers with Harvey's metal binder paperclip."

"Fuck, that's a brilliant idea!" Stanley chimed in, his eyes gleaming with wicked excitement. "Remember how her body was shaking in pain with the clamp on her tiny little clit? That would... Damn! That tight little hole would be an even better cock-milking tunnel."

"Her screams alone would make it worth it," Theo added, grinning sadistically.

"Doesn't she look so fucking hot like this?" Cliff asked as he watched Bernard's powerful thrusts. "Her perfect ass bouncing, her feet aching with each step on the gravel... I bet she's never been this desperate and broken before."

"Nothing quite like taking a beautiful, proud, perfect young thing like her and making her want to suffer for our pleasure," another man agreed, his eyes glued to my trembling body.

As another man positioned himself behind me and began to ram into my ass mercilessly, pushing my feet further down the gravel path, tears streamed down my face from the unbearable pain in my anus, my battered feet, and my scalp.

Despite this torment, my mind traveled back to the potential agony of having my clit clamped with a binder clip while being savagely pounded like this. The thought filled me with dread yet, at the same time, an odd sense of excitement. I kept wondering how fuckin' intense it would be and how much better it would be for my god—these men's old cocks.

And then, inside me, I became sad. My owners had moved on from that suggestion as if it would be too sadistic even for them.

"Please," I whimpered between ragged breaths, "next time... use the binder clip on my clit." My voice was barely audible, but the men around me seemed to perk up, their eyes widening in intrigued delight.

"Did she just..." Charles started, his voice trailing off as he glanced at the others for confirmation.

"Did she really just ask for that?" Wilfred chimed in, grinning wickedly.

"Fuck, she's even more twisted than we thought!" Theo exclaimed, rubbing his hands together in anticipation.

"Are you sure about that, baby girl?" Harvey asked, raising one eyebrow and studying my tear-streaked face. "You want us to clamp that tender little clit of yours, all while we continue to pound your ass on the gravel?"

I nodded frantically, desperation seeping into my voice. "Do you... Does it make your cocks hard to think about it?"

"Well, fuck ya! But..."

"Yes, yes!" I insisted, "Please do it. Hurt me more. Your cocks deserve a better massage."

Meanwhile, Edgar had taken over, gripping my hips tightly as he thrust into my abused asshole. My feet howled in agony as they scraped against the gravel with each violent movement, but I couldn't deny the dark thrill coursing through me at the prospect of the additional torture I had requested.

"Damn, Delisha, I never would've pegged you as such a pain slut when we met you at Miami airport yesterday," Cliff remarked, clearly amused by my perverse request. "But hey, if you're game..."

"Let me get this straight," Theo interjected, a sinister smile playing on his lips. "You want us to clamp your clit with a brutal binder clip while we fuck your ass, and you're going to beg for it?"

"Y-yes," I stammered. "I'll beg you. For you. And your cocks." The words felt like a surrender but also a declaration of my own twisted desires. "Don't you guys hate clits?"

The men around us exchanged glances, their expressions a mix of shock and arousal. They had never met someone like me, willing to do anything to pleasure their cocks.

"Jesus Christ," muttered Theo, his eyes wide as he watched my ass being mercilessly pounded. "She's really begging for this."

"Can't say I've ever seen anything like it," Francis chimed in, clearly excited by the prospect of seeing me in even more pain. "But, fuck... My cock is hard for sure!"

I braced myself against the rough gravel as another man drove his hard rod into my ass, relishing in the dual sensations of pain and pleasure coursing through me. As he grunted and thrust, my craving for extreme sexual pain grew stronger with each hurtful step forward.

"Please, promise to use the binder clip on my clit next time," I whimper, barely able to form coherent words as he pounded into me relentlessly. The men watching us exchanged incredulous glances before their eyes narrowed with predatory hunger.

"Fuck, Delisha, you're such a depraved little whore," Fred chimes in, his hand idly stroking his thickening cock as he watches the violent coupling happening on the gravel trail. "What kind of sick bitch begs for her clit to be tortured like that?"

"It's for you," I whispered in pain, "don't you hate cock teasing blondes?"

"God damn," Victor mutters, shaking his head in disbelief. "Don't worry, then, we'll make sure you get exactly what you're asking for... or more!"

"Fuck, this girl is kinky as hell," a man murmured, his eyes fixed on my tortured body.

Eventually, the 14th man was done beating my ass, and I was on the verge of collapse, my body battered and abused by the group of men who had taken turns pounding my ass on the rough gravel trail. The sensation had been excruciating, but the desire for more pain only grew within me.

So, after what felt like hours of torturous walking, they allowed me to stop. Gasping for breath, I collapsed on the grass on all fours with nausea. My feet throbbing with pain, and my body still quivering from the relentless abuse, I reached down and grazed my fingertips over my swollen clit. The touch sent a jolt of pleasure mixed with trepidation through me as I anticipated what they would do to me later that week.

"Your parents must be so proud," a man chimed in, chuckling darkly. "Their precious little girl, such a pain slut."

"Actually," I confessed, feeling a strange sense of pride, "my Mom and Dad know all about it. I will tell them about this trip. They always said I had an unusually high tolerance for sexual pain. But I think it's more than just tolerance... it's a craving."

"Is that so?" one of the men mused, intrigued by my admission. "Then I guess we're going to have to give you exactly what you crave, aren't we? More pain to share with Mommy and Daddy?"

The crude comments continued, each one stirring a potent cocktail of fear and desire within me. I knew that the worst was yet to come—and I couldn't wait.

16

I Was Offered To 17 Old Cocks as The Sex Pet of The Whole Dive Resort

I lay crumpled on the grass beside the gravel trail, my tender feet, abused butthole, and aching scalp screaming for relief. The 14 old men who owned me had just taken turns violating my ass as they forced me to walk the rough path.

They then gathered around me like well-fed vultures waiting for their next feast, their lewd laughter echoing in my ears.

"Her tight little butthole clenched every time she stepped on a sharp stone," one of the men recounted, his voice dripping with depraved excitement. "It was like her ass was milking my cock!"

"No kidding!" another chimed in, smirking down at me. "Never felt anything like it before."

Their words made me proud. These men had used me, pushed me past my limits, and all I could think about was how much more I wanted. How much more I needed.

“Her ass tightened so much around me, thought I was gonna implode!"

"Damn right, her ass clenched around my cock like a vice every time she stepped on the gravel," one man said, his eyes raking over my naked form with shameless hunger.

"Made me shoot my load faster than ever before," another chimed in, smirking at me as if I were nothing more than a cock sleeve for their pleasure.

I often explained to friends and people reading my sex confessions how much I want to be just like a cock-pleasuring tool – something men use to masturbate instead of a pocket pussy. And these men were doing just that. All of them. They didn't care about my bare feet hurting on the gravel. They simply wanted their cock to be milked by my butthole, and gravel on my feet was simply a button to activate the milking feature in the fuck doll's ass. And I fuckin' loved it!

Two men from the group of 17 other divers approached, their curiosity piqued by the scene before them. Harvey was quick to fill them in on what they'd missed. My face flushed with shame and arousal as I heard him recount, in explicit detail, how they'd all taken turns pounding my ass while forcing me to walk on the gravel trail. The way he described each thrust, each grunt of pleasure, and every tightening of my abused butthole made me ache for more, even as I knew I should be repulsed.

"Damn," one of the newcomers breathed, his disappointment evident. "Wish we could've gotten in on that action."

"Didn't you hear at lunch?" Harvey asked, genuinely surprised. "You're welcome to use our little sex pet here whenever you want. Let's say... She's like a piece of furniture or a toy included with the resort."

"Like a long chair by the pool! Free use," another one added. "If she's free, grab her."

A sinister grin spread across the newcomers' faces, and I could see the wheels turning in their heads as they considered the possibilities. I braced myself for whatever depraved act they would come up with next, my body trembling with anticipation.

"Tell you what," Harvey proposed, now addressing the whole group of 14 men owning my body. "Why don't we walk her around and offer her to each of the other guys in turn? Break the ice, so to speak. Some of them might be shy about taking advantage of our sweet sex pet here."

“Slave,” I corrected him. “Sex slave.”

As they conspired, my mind raced with excitement. The thought of being paraded around like a prostitute, offered to each man in turn, made me wet. I felt like the luckiest girl on earth!

The two newcomers were eager to volunteer to start the process. But after the brutal pounding my ass and feet had endured on the gravel trail, there was no way I could walk. The solution: they removed my handcuffs, and then four of the men grabbed my ankles and wrists, hoisting me up like a piece of meat.

"Let's get this little fuck toy to the cabin," one of them grunted as they carried me along, my naked body stretched and wobbling between them. As we moved through the tropical paradise, surrounded by palm trees and ocean breezes, I reveled in the sensation of being utterly exposed and vulnerable. My submissive heart soared as I was carried like a piece of meat to be offered to so many old men.

Upon reaching the cabin, I felt the cool air of the cabin brush against my naked, vulnerable body as the four men released their grip on my wrists and ankles, allowing my battered form to crumple onto the soft bed. The two strangers gazed down at me, their eyes hungrily devouring my every curve, their hands twitching with the urge to claim what they had been promised.

"Remember," one of the men carrying me warned them just before leaving, "make sure she begs for it. Don't give her a break."

"Once you're done using her," another chimed in, "bring her back to the pool on her leash. We've got big plans for the rest of the afternoon."

The crude instructions made me shiver, my body aching for more punishment.

"Look at her," one of them growled, his voice thick with desire. "Isn't she just a perfect little fuckdoll?"

"Absolutely beautiful," the other agreed, reaching out to gently trace a fingertip over my swollen nipples, causing me to shudder involuntarily. "Such a pretty piece of ass for us to play with."

"Please," I begged, parting my trembling thighs to reveal my dripping core, desperate for them to fill me with their cocks. "I need you inside me. Just take me and use me however you want."

A devilish grin spread across the man's face as he watched me squirm with need. "You heard the girl," he told his friend, positioning himself behind me as I got on all fours. Without any further warning, he rammed his hard cock into my tight pussy, drawing a strangled moan from my lips as he began to pound me mercilessly.

"Open that filthy mouth of yours," the other man commanded, guiding his erect member toward my eager lips. I didn't hesitate to comply, wrapping my lips around his shaft and sucking him like a god would deserve. Have I mentioned that old cocks are my god?

"Be rougher with me," I managed to gasp between thrusts, the sensation of both my holes being filled driving me wild with lust. "Please, punish this little blonde cock tease."

"Fuck, you're such a dirty slut," the man in my pussy groaned, gripping my hips tightly as he slammed into me even harder. "With a fuckin' tight pussy!"

After having gotten my ass beaten by 14 cocks, it was refreshing to feel a rod inside my real cock-pleasuring tunnel while my knees were comfortably resting on a mattress. His forceful thrusts sent intense waves of pleasure crashing through me, mingling with the pain to create a heady cocktail that left me dizzy and desperate for more.

"Make her scream," the other man urged, his own thrusts becoming more forceful as he buried himself deep within my throat. The sensation of being so thoroughly used and abused was intoxicating, pushing me closer and closer to the edge of orgasm. But I didn't want to climax. I feel more like a fuck doll if I never get an orgasm. Ever.

"Please. Push my head down further," I gasped, my voice muffled by the man's cock in my mouth. He obliged, gripping my hair and forcing his throbbing member deeper into my throat until my top lip pressed against his belly and my bottom lip grazed his balls.

"Rougher," I panted when the man in my mouth allowed me a second to breathe. "Please... beat my tight pussy like you always wanted to punish a blonde cock tease."

My plea seemed to fuel their lust as they both increased their pace, pounding my body with raw, animalistic force. And as they continued to fuck me mercilessly, I reveled in the crude, violent language they used to describe my naked form. It was degrading, but it only served to heighten my desire for submission. Their words filled my mind with filthy images, making me hungrier for their cocks and the painful pleasure they inflicted upon me.

"Look at this tight little cunt," the man behind me grunted, slapping my ass hard enough to send a stinging wave through my flesh. "She wants it so bad, doesn't she?"

"Filthy slut needs her holes filled," the other agreed, gripping my hair and forcing my head back onto his rock-hard dick. "It's her lucky day!"

"Can't... can't believe how tight she is," the man behind me panted, his thrusts growing more erratic as his level of excitement increased. "Gonna... gonna fuck her all week."

"Damn right," the one in my mouth agreed, pulling out just enough to let me gasp for air before shoving himself back down my throat. "Best little fuck toy we've ever had."

"Please," I begged, my words muffled by the thick cock filling my mouth, "push it deeper... I can take it."

The man receiving my eager blowjob smirked and grabbed a fistful of my blonde hair. As he pushed my head down, his swollen member slid further into my throat until my top lip kissed his belly, and my bottom lip was on his balls. My body trembled in response to the intense sensation, but I craved more.

"Keep going," I gasped when he let me up for air, my eyes watering from the effort. "Hold me down; choke me until I tap your leg."

He did as I asked, pushing my head back onto his throbbing cock, relentlessly forcing it down my throat as I struggled for a breath. My hand rested on his thigh, ready to tap out when I couldn't take it any longer.

"Fuck, how can she breathe like that?" The man fucking my pussy from behind grunted in disbelief, his hips slamming against my buttocks with brutal force.

"Never seen anything like it," the man in my mouth muttered, clearly impressed by my ability to hold my breath and pleasure him simultaneously.

But soon enough, the man pounding my pussy couldn't resist the temptation to see for himself. So they switched positions, and I eagerly welcomed his cock into my throat, reveling in the chance to be abused in such a deliciously filthy way.

"Jesus Christ," he groaned as I took him deep, my nose buried in his pubic hair. "This slut's a fucking pro."

Feeling their admiration and desire for my submissive display only fueled how proud I am of my abilities to please cock-carrying beasts. I continued to choke on his cock, determined to show them just how far I was willing to go for their pleasure.

"Can't... believe this," the man now behind me panted, his grip on my hips tightening as he rammed into my pussy with animalistic hunger. My body shook with each thrust, but the pain mingled with perverse satisfaction as I offered myself up to these two men.

"God, she's amazing," the one in my mouth moaned when I finally tapped his leg, signaling it was time to release me. He reluctantly pulled out, allowing me to catch my breath as I coughed and gasped for air, a string of drool connecting my lips to his wet shaft.

"Never had a babe like her before," the man fucking my pussy grunted, his movements growing more erratic as he neared his climax. "She's the perfect doll."

As the men continued to pound me, one in my mouth and the other in my love canal, I suddenly realized that they hadn't used condoms. The realization sent a thrill down my spine – it was wrong, but the sensation of their raw cocks inside me was too intoxicating to resist. The skin of a cock on my tongue is one of life's greatest pleasures, and I need sperm in my belly to live. That's all I intended to eat this week. And a girl needs to be fed.

But it was wrong. So, do what I say, not what I do, and use a condom.

"Fuck, she's so tight," the man fucking my pussy groaned, his grip on my hips bruising as he slammed into me with abandon.

"Can't wait to fill her up," the man in my mouth grunted, his hands tangled in my hair as he forced his cock deeper down my throat.

I knew it wasn't safe – the 14 men who owned me had been health tested before the trip, but these two were strangers. They'd been told they could use my body, but only with protection. Still, I couldn't bring myself to care. My craving for their sperm, my insatiable hunger to be a spermivore, overrode any sense of caution.

Besides, these old married men probably hadn't had sex in a long time, I mused, the thought driving me wild as I willingly submitted to their depraved desires. I wanted their seed, wanted to taste it and feel it filling me up, sealing my fate as their willing fuck toy.

"God, I'm gonna cum," the man in my ass announced, his thrusts becoming more erratic.

"Me too," the one in my mouth added, his grip on my hair tightening.

They both reached their climax almost simultaneously. The man in my pussy pulled out just in time to spray his load all over my back while the one in my mouth held me down, forcing me to swallow every drop of his release. I choked and coughed but didn't dare tap out – I wanted every last bit of his essence.

"Jesus Christ," one of them panted as they finally let me up for air. "That was fucking incredible."

"Unbelievable," the other agreed, his eyes glazed with lust as he stared down at my cum-covered body.

They grabbed my leash and led me back to the pool area, naked and dripping with their seed. They couldn't stop talking about how amazing I was – how tight my pussy was, how well I took their cocks in my mouth – and how much they wanted to keep pounding me all week long.

You may think I am weird, but it is an intense pleasure for me to hear old men satisfied after they've used my body. I won't be young forever, so now is the time to make old men happy with a young body, tight pussy, willing throat, and firm boobs.

The sensation of being led by a leash, naked and covered in men's cum, along a path surrounded by palm trees on a tropical paradise island was pure ecstasy. As they handed the leash over to one of my owners, I felt like a prized possession – something that these men were proud to have control over.

"God, you wouldn't believe how tight her pussy is," one of them boasted, grinning at the others. "And she can deepthroat like a fucking champ."

The man who had taken my leash, Victor, smirked as he tugged it slightly, forcing me to step closer to him. The other men gathered around, ogling my cum-covered body.

I felt a mixture of shame and arousal at their words. This was exactly what I wanted – to be an object for their lust, a toy for their amusement. My pussy throbbed with need, aching for more attention. I needed these other 15 men to use the dive resort sex pet. Now. I needed them now.

And the owners of my body didn't disappoint me.

They insisted that every other man at the pool grab my leash, drag me to their cabin, and make me beg to be abused. And then, once all the men at the pool had dipped their cocks in the blonde bimbo, my owners walked around the resort, parading my nude body, looking for any man in the group of 17 who hadn't yet given me a beating with their male rod. They wanted every man at the resort to break the ice so they would be comfortable abusing me for the rest of the week.

Some of the men weren't interested at first, but my owners

convinced them that using the resort sex slave was not cheating on their wives more than masturbating with tissue paper. And the argument worked. Men are easily convinced when their penis is erect!

So by the end of the afternoon on the first day of our week-long dive vacation, all 14 and 17 cocks had pounded the young blonde nude chick. In the process, I got 8 loads of sperm in my belly, which was much less than planned.

I wanted to ingest at least one liter of male semen over the week and had planned to achieve it by sucking 14 cocks, three times a day all week. On Sunday afternoon, after 24 hours at the dive resort, I had so far only been fed 39 loads. To be on schedule, I needed another 29 loads before the end of the day on Sunday.

Being fed semen on a regular basis was the reason I had organized this trip in the first place. Most people don't comprehend it, but sperm, to me, is the most delicious candy, and I can't get enough of it. It's comforting to have in my mouth, like hot milk.

Yet, I couldn't complain about how the week got off track because these men were giving me something else I've always craved and that so few men are comfortable doing for me.

And I wasn't in charge anymore – not even of my body. My owners would decide if and when I would be fed.

Dinnertime came quickly, and my naked body was once more displayed on a table as we did at lunchtime, only this time, I was not gagged. The men seemed to enjoy making me beg continuously. The butt plug and handcuffs were also gone – lost along the trail or in a cabin at one point in the afternoon. Therefore, I could be on display in the standard submissive pose: on my knees, legs apart to expose my young tight pussy, hands on my thighs with palm up, back arched to further display my young firm tits, and eyes down, never looking up unless asked to.

What a sight! Thirty-one old men were having their meal, sitting on comfortable chairs, while I, a nude young blonde woman, was kneeling on a hard surface with my legs spread wide, revealing my tight, tender pussy. Each of these elderly men had his penis inside me at some point during the day. I was proud of being able to do such a thing. They owned me in every way possible – they even confiscated my passport and ID papers, along with all of my clothing, which they threw away. I had no idea when or how I would be able to leave the island.

And then I began to entertain the idea of becoming a sex slave, permanently stationed at the dive resort. What if I never went back home? What if I stayed at the resort, ready for service—naked—all year round? I would need to plead with customers for access to a cabin at night. Without their consent, I'd be forced to sleep outdoors on the beach. I would depend on men's semen for nutrition. The picture of me as a permanently enslaved sex object aroused my desires.

Yes, I know, I'm twisted! And that fantasy will most likely never happen. But I was having the time of my life!

17

I Begged 31 Old Men To Torture My Clitoris To Entertain Them & Massage Their Cocks

I remained on my knees on a hard table in front of all 31 old men who had come to the dive resort for a week of scuba diving. I could feel their lecherous eyes devouring my young, nude female body and felt powerless to protect myself. My legs were splayed open to reveal the depths of my tight pussy, offering them a view that ignited a desire in their veins. As instructed, I rested my hands on the softness of my thighs, palms up. And I arched my back, as ordered, thrusting out my young, firm breasts as if they were there for the taking. Never did I dare look up from beneath my lashes until they beckoned me to do so, for then I was fully under their control.

The 14 old men I traveled with had broken me in less than 24 hours, beating me into total submission, and claimed full ownership of my body. And then, they shared their sex slave with the other 17 men at the resort for the week.

As I kneeled there, completely vulnerable and exposed, I could feel the weight of their gazes on me. The air was thick with anticipation and lust as they eagerly discussed my erotic submission in crude, explicit language.

"Look at that perfect little cunt," one man said, motioning towards my exposed pussy. "Just begging to be filled."

"Her tits are so perky, damn! I want to bring them home with me," another chimed in, his eyes devouring my breasts.

"Can't wait to see her suck some more of my cock," a third one added, smirking at my display.

Their comments fueled my submissive desires, and I reveled in being their object of lust. I knew they saw me as a sex object, something to be used and enjoyed for their pleasure, and I loved it.

I remembered that I hadn't eaten dinner—but that didn't matter. My hunger was for semen, not plain ordinary food, and soon enough, these elderly men would satisfy my craving.

One man leaned forward, placing his rough hand on my inner thigh. "I can't believe this little slut took all of us today. She's so tiny, yet she handled our pounding like a fucking champ. 31 times!"

"Her tight holes just kept milking our cocks," another chimed in, grinning at the memory of my body clenching around him. "She's built to be fucked and used by us old bastards."

A member of the group of 17, curiosity piqued, asked the 14 men about the story they had heard earlier. "So what's this we've been hearing about her walking on gravel while you guys fucked her ass?"

My owners grinned proudly, eager to boast about their devious exploits. "Oh yeah, that was something else," one of them began. "We made her walk on gravel, barefoot, while we plowed her tight little asshole. Every time her feet landed on those sharp stones, her butthole would clench around our cocks, giving us the most amazing massage and milking we've ever had."

"Her whimpers and cries only made it hotter," another added, his eyes gleaming with cruel satisfaction. "Seeing such a sexy young thing hurting and crying while being brutally fucked... It was the perfect mix of... Erotic show!"

My face flushed, a mix of shame and arousal coursing through me as I listened to them recount their depraved acts. Despite the humiliation, I couldn't deny that their words stirred something deep within me, feeding my masochistic desires. I wanted more of it.

Another chimed in, his voice dripping with lustful recollection. "Her tears streaming down her face, her body trembling in pain... It made my cock so hard... It was easy to pound that tight ass."

My cheeks burned with humiliation, but I couldn't deny the way my body responded to their words, my nipples tightening and a familiar ache growing between my thighs.

"Invite us next time you do that, at least to watch," one of the men from the group of 17 said, eager to join in on the degrading spectacle. The others nodded in agreement, their eyes raking over my exposed flesh hungrily.

"Actually, we've got something even better planned for you," the leader of the group of 14 declared, smirking at me wickedly. "Come with us to the beach right now. Trust me, you won't want to miss it."

My body trembled with anticipation as the group of 14 men led us all toward the beach, my naked form being pulled along by a leash attached to my collar. The salty sea breeze caressed my exposed skin, making my nipples harden even more.

As we made our way to the beach, they ordered me to walk barefoot in the middle of the gravel trail. My feet were tender and delicate, each step sending jolts of pain up my legs as the sharp stones bit into my soft flesh. My buttocks clenched reflexively with each painful step, providing the men with the show they wanted.

"You were right! Look at how her perfect little ass tightens as she walks on those stones," someone from the group of 17 observed, his voice thick with arousal.

"Damn, that's one sexy girl," another added, his gaze locked on my tormented form.

Meanwhile, the men walked comfortably on the grass beside the trail, wearing sandals and smirking at my predicament. The contrast was stark—all of them clothed and comfortable, with their feet well protected, while I was naked, barefoot, and in pain. Their laughter and jeers filled the air, mingling with my stifled whimpers of distress.

My heart pounded as one of my owners grabbed me roughly by the arm, forcing me to stop. “You know what, girl? You’re just a cock tease that deserves to be punished. You need to beg for this pain,” he growled, his breath hot and heavy against my ear.

“Please,” I whispered, my voice trembling with a mixture of fear and excitement. “Please force me to walk barefoot on the gravel. It’s what I deserve.” A part of me couldn’t believe that I was actually uttering those words, but my body responded with a shudder of anticipation.

“Ha! Good girl,” he sneered, giving my ass a hard slap. The other men laughed, their eyes filled with lust as they watched me submit.

“Say it louder,” another man demanded, his voice dripping with authority. “Beg for your punishment.”

“Please!” I cried out louder this time. “Make me walk barefoot on the gravel! I’m just a cock tease!”

“And?” the man insisted.

“I’m... My only purpose in life is to be entertainment for all of you!”

The men in the group of 17 stared at me, their cocks visibly straining against their pants as they took in the sight of my submissiveness along my vulnerable, exposed young female body. They murmured amongst themselves, clearly aroused by the raw display of dominance from their peers.

“Look at her,” one of them said, his voice thick with desire. “Her tight little ass clenches so deliciously with every step. So delicate... Fragile... Hot! She’s a hottie!”

“Fuck, yeah,” another agreed, his eyes glued to my agonized movements. “There’s something so fucking hot about watching her suffer like this. She might be a tease, but she’s putting on one hell of a show.”

These old men were appreciative of what I was doing, and that was all I needed to keep going. Since I started exploring my sexuality as a teenager, I've craved using my naked body to provide entertainment to old men, as long as they appreciate the effort.

So I continued to walk along the gravel trail, each step sending sharp jolts of pain through my body. My cheeks flushed with a mix of embarrassment and satisfaction as I witnessed how much my pain and humiliation were turning these men on.

"You like it, guys? Such a tight little ass," one of the men from the group of 14 chuckled, his hand reaching out to give it a rough slap, which made me yelp and sent shivers down my spine. "Just wait till you see what we have in store for our little blonde pet."

The sound of waves crashing on the shore filled the air as we arrived at the beach. The sun was setting, casting an orange glow over everything and making my sweaty, glistening skin look even more enticing. The men ogled my helpless form, their crude comments fueling my arousal even further.

"God, I loved burying my face in her tits this afternoon," one of the men from the group of 17 mused.

"And they taste as good as they look, don't they?" Victor responded, grinning wickedly as he glanced at my breasts. I could feel their eyes on me, tearing away any last shred of dignity I had left.

As I stood there, exposed and humiliated, I knew I craved this treatment. My body was theirs, my mind consumed by the need to submit.

"Please," I whispered, my eyes downcast as I addressed the men who owned me. "Use me however you want. I'm here to serve you."

"Good girl," Harvey said, giving my ass another rough smack. "By the end of tonight, everybody will know exactly what you're meant for."

As six men from the group of 14 led me into the ocean, I could feel the hungry eyes of the other men on the beach. My naked body was exposed and vulnerable, my breasts bouncing with each step as the waves crashed around my thighs. The water was cool against my skin, washing away the remnants of their lust that still clung to my body.

"Look at her," one of the men from the group of 17 said, his voice laced with crude arousal. "Like a sexy little mermaid on a leash."

"Wait 'til you see what's next," Theo replied, smirking at the anticipation on the men's faces.

I felt the hands of the six old men on my body, rubbing and scrubbing at my flesh, cleaning me of the leftover sperm. Their fingers dug into my soft skin, gripping my hips, my ass, and my breasts as they worked to wash me clean. They were washing their pet! And each touch reminded me of my place, my role in society as a young blonde.

My mind wandered to the fact that this was my first contact with the ocean since arriving at the dive resort. Despite my love for scuba diving and the sea, the group of 14 decided that I didn't deserve to explore the depths of the ocean during this trip. They had deemed me a naughty cock tease, unworthy of such pleasures, and my punishment was to satisfy their most twisted desires for the rest of the week.

The conflict raged within me; I ached to be used by these men to satisfy their carnal hunger, but my love for the ocean and scuba diving threatened to overpower it. I craved the freedom of diving beneath the surface, exploring the mysteries of the deep blue sea. But as those rough hands continued to cleanse me, my desire to submit seemed to grow stronger.

"Tell us how much you need this, baby girl," Harvey commanded, pulling me closer to him by the leash.

"Please," I whimpered, feeling the weight of their gazes on my trembling form. "I need this. I need to be used by you all."

"Such a good little whore," Stanley murmured approvingly, his fingers pinching one of my nipples as they continued to scrub away at my body.

After the six men finished washing me, leaving me shivering with anticipation, they dragged me back to the beach, my body still glistening with seawater. The men in the group of 17 couldn't take their eyes off me, and I could feel my cheeks burning with embarrassment. But deep down, I knew that I craved this attention—to be the object of their filthy desires.

"Damn, look at her now," one man from the group of 17 said. "Her hair all wet like that, clinging to her perfect tits... She's even more beautiful."

"Fuck, yeah," another man agreed, rubbing his crotch as he stared at me. "I'd love to run my fingers through those wet locks while I pound her tight little pussy."

As the men continued to comment on my appearance, I couldn't help but feel a sick sense of satisfaction. I loved being their dirty fantasy.

"Alright, Delisha," Theo said, tightening his grip on my leash. "Tell these men what your purpose is for this week."

Swallowing hard, I forced the words out. "I'm here to serve you, to pleasure you in any way you desire. I'm your sex pet. And your cock is a god to be worshipped."

"Good girl," Harvey praised, grinning wickedly. "Now beg us to use you more. Show these men how desperate you are for our cocks."

Feeling the weight of their expectant stares, I dropped to my knees in the sand, the warm grains pressing into my skin. "Please," I whispered, trying to ignore the shame that threatened to choke me. "Please use me more. I need your cocks inside me, using me like the slutty bitch I am."

"See?" Fred boasted to the group of 17, who were watching with a mixture of shock and lust.

With each degrading order and filthy comment, I found myself sinking deeper into my role as a non-human sex object. And despite the turmoil raging within me, a part of me knew that this was exactly where I belonged—on my knees, begging to be beaten by godly cocks.

My owners laughed and jeered as they continued to entertain their audience. I could feel their eyes on me, scanning my soaked body like a piece of meat. One man from the group of 17 said, "That little slut's butthole must've been tight around your cocks when you fucked her on that gravel trail."

"Damn right it was," Theo responded, smirking at me. "But did our cocks get the milking they deserved? Let's hear what our cock tease here thinks."

"Delisha," Harvey said, his voice cold and commanding, "did our cocks deserve better than what you gave us on the gravel trail?"

My cheeks flushed with humiliation as I looked up at him. "Yes," I whispered, feeling the weight of their stares. "Your cocks deserved better."

"Tell them why," Cliff demanded, grabbing a fistful of my wet hair and forcing me to look at the group of 17. "Tell them why you deserved to suffer on that trail and why it was not enough."

"Because... because I've been a cock tease for years," I admitted, choking back tears. "And because young blondes like me are pretentious little things who need to be put in our place."

"Good girl," Victor praised, releasing my hair. "Now bow and apologize to us for not giving us a better cock massage while we fucked your ass."

"Please forgive me," I begged, pressing my forehead against the warm sand. "I'm so sorry I didn't do a better job when you fucked my ass. I promise to make it up to you."

Theo stepped forward and smirked down at me. "You've begged for forgiveness, but now, we want you to beg for a chance to do better than those pathetic cock massages you gave us on the gravel trail."

Heat rushed to my cheeks, and I struggled to meet his eyes, knowing exactly what was expected of me and how much it would hurt. "Please," I whispered hoarsely, "give me a chance to make it up to you, to provide better cock massages for the pleasure of my god, your cocks."

"Ha, look at her," Harvey sneered, gesturing at my submissive form. "She knows she fucked up and can't wait to take our cocks again."

"Alright, Delisha," Charles chimed in, his tone mocking, "if you want to prove yourself, tell us how you think you can make your tight little butthole clench harder to milk our cocks better?"

My stomach twisted into knots; they were leading me to the abyss, but I had asked for it earlier in the afternoon. It was my idea! I wanted their cocks to be worshipped even more. The eyes of both groups of men were glued to my lips. "You... You could try torturing my clit," I mumbled, not daring to look up at them.

The men from the group of 17 stared at me with wide-eyed fascination, clearly impressed by my debasing suggestions. Their lustful gazes roamed over my naked body as if they were already fantasizing about what they could do to me.

"Alright, Delisha," said Francis, one of my owners who had been enjoying my torment. "We want ideas for how we can torture that pretty little clit of yours to make your tight asshole clench around our cocks. And you better beg us nicely."

"You... you could put a binder paperclip on my clit while you fuck my ass. The pain would force me to clench around you," I stammered, then added quickly, "Please... I want to give you the best cock massage possible."

"Did you hear that?" Charles asked the group of 17, clearly proud of the sex pet. "She's begging for us to put a fucking binder clip on her clit."

"Damn, she either loves pain or she really wants to pleasure cocks," one of the men from the group of 17 said, clearly disbelieving.

"I think she sees old men's cocks as some sort of a god for her," one of my owners answered, laughing.

"Prove it to them, Delisha," Stanley ordered. "Convince these men that you're serious about giving us all a better cock massage by torturing your clit."

"Please," I pleaded, my voice cracking with desperation. "I need to give you the best possible pleasure because your cocks deserve it, and the best way for me to do that is by hurting my clit. You deserve it."

"Damn, she's the ultimate fuck doll," one of the men from the group of 17 muttered, finally seeming convinced by my desperate pleas.

"Alright, Delisha, since you want it so badly," Theo said with a wicked grin, "we'll make sure you feel every ounce of pain necessary to worship our cocks properly this week. Starting tonight, with that binder clip you begged for."

"Thank you," I whispered, trembling in anticipation and fear but also with a growing hunger for the pain and humiliation that would remind me of my place as a sex toy, with my clit being nothing but a button to activate cock milking.

18

31 Old Men Tortured My Clit to Get The Ultimate Cock Massage From My Butthole at a Tropical Dive Resort

I found myself on the warm, soft sand of a tropical beach, completely nude, with 31 old men standing around me in their bathing suits, their eyes ravenous as they hungrily devoured my naked body with their lustful gazes. The leash attached to my collar was a symbol of my submission to their desires, a guarantee their male needs would be satisfied on that beach.

Cocks were my gods, and serving them was my purpose.

Earlier in the day, the 14 men who owned me had pounded my ass while making me walk barefoot on gravel, my butthole clenching automatically at each painful step, massaging their cocks in the process and driving them wild. But now, I wanted to prove that I could do even better for them. I lowered my eyes, my voice dripping with desperate need.

"Please," I whimpered, my naked body shining under the moonlight as I knelt in front of my masters and owners. My hands were clasped together, my eyes pleading with the men surrounding me. "I can do better than before. I want to give you even more pleasure." As I spoke, I could feel their eyes roaming over my exposed flesh, lingering on my full breasts and the curve of my hips.

"Tell us how," one man demanded, his voice thick with lust.

"Put your cocks in my ass," I moaned, "and then snap a hard binder paperclip on my clit. It'll make my butthole clench even tighter around your cock. Please," I begged, my face flushed with arousal, "You deserve all the pleasure you can get."

The men couldn't resist their animalistic desires any longer. Surveying the beach, they found a perfect spot where the sand sloped gently down to the water's edge. Eager hands molded a small mound of sand, shaping it into a makeshift cushion for my ass.

"Put your ass on this pile, babe," Theo commanded, his voice thick with lust. "It'll be the perfect height for us to fuck you while we're on our knees."

I obeyed without hesitation, positioning my body over the sand mound and lowering myself onto it. My butthole was now raised, perfectly poised and exposed for their eager cocks. My head tipped back, sinking lower into the sand, emphasizing how that part of my nude body didn't matter to them. I was just a butthole to use and a clit to torture. And I had to make both readily available to them.

Harvey stepped forward, his hard cock already out as he knelt between my spread legs. The sight of his engorged member so close to my vulnerable hole sent shivers of anticipation down my spine.

"It's my paperclip, so I go first," he announced.

"Now," I rasped. "I'm all yours."

He thrust his hard rod into my ass, and I screamed in ecstasy as a new pain bloomed inside me. They were going to break me, fuck me raw, on this beach, and I would worship them for it.

"Open those pretty pussy lips for me, Delisha," Harvey growled, his eyes locked onto my sex. "Push the hood aside, and let me see that tiny clit of yours."

With trembling fingers, I did as he asked, spreading my outer lips wide and revealing my swollen clit. As I held it exposed, Harvey smirked and added, "Now beg for that clamp, baby girl."

"Please, Daddy," I whimpered, a mixture of fear and arousal making my voice shake. "Snap that hard binder paper clip on my clit.

Your cock is my god. I'm just a blonde cock tease that deserves to be beaten."

As those crude, degrading words left my lips, the air seemed to hum with tension. The men's lustful eyes bore into me, their cocks aching to claim and dominate my young, willing body.

"Please, Daddy," I rasped, my voice hoarse from the continuous begging. "One clit hurting for 31 worshipped hard cocks. It's worth it!" My body trembled with a familiar mix of excitement and fear coursing through me. Harvey making me wait was more painful than anything else, I thought at the moment.

"Such a filthy little bitch," Harvey growled approvingly. "Alright, babe. You've earned it."

With a swift, merciless motion, Harvey snapped the hard binder paper clip onto my throbbing clit. The intense, searing pain shot through me like a bolt of lightning, making me scream and arch my back off the sand.

I gotta tell you, clit torture is the best exercise for abs. And I wouldn't have it any other way.

The men around me let out raucous laughter and crude remarks, their cocks twitching at the sight of my suffering.

"God, look at her squirm," one of the men in the group of 17 cackled, his eyes glued to the spot where the metal teeth of the clip bit into my tender flesh. "She's a real pain slut, isn't she?"

"Absolutely beautiful," another one agreed as he watched my body convulse under the relentless torment. "Can't wait to fuck that tight ass of hers while she's in agony."

My body shook uncontrollably as the sharp pain from the binder clip on my clit kept sending shockwaves through me. Tears streamed down my face, but that only seemed to excite the men around me even more. Their laughter filled the air, a chorus of crude delight at my torment.

"Fuck, just look at her," Theo barked out between laughs, his eyes raking over my writing form. "Never thought I'd see the day when a perfect blonde babe would be begging for this kind of punishment."

"Dumb blonde, what do you expect?" a cruel man observed.

The others chimed in with their own lewd comments, each one more depraved than the last. As their words washed over me, I felt a twisted and intense sense of satisfaction in knowing that I was the reason for 31 old cocks to be harder than they probably had been in a long time.

They didn't need Viagra with me.

"Her ass is clenching so tight, just like she's trying to squeeze the life out of my cock," Harvey grunted, his hips thrusting wildly as he continued to pound into me. "I don't know what it is about that binder clip, but damn if she isn't milking me harder than ever before."

He was right—the pain shooting through my clit with each heartbeat triggered involuntary spasms in my ass, gripping Harvey's cock relentlessly. And the truth was, I had never experienced anything that intense before. Earlier this year, I thought I had reached the ultimate in clit torturing, but this was bringing it up a notch. Would I ever find my pain limit?

And despite the agony, or perhaps because of it, my need for their brutal domination grew stronger by the second. I knew I would be sharing this sexual experience with you guys, and knowing your cocks would also get hard motivated me even more.

"Please, don't stop," I gasped out, surprising even myself with the raw desperation in my voice. "My body is only good at worshipping cocks."

"Damn, she's greedy," Stanley marveled, his hand wrapped tightly around his own erection as he watched the scene unfold. "Maybe next dive trip, we should have a hundred men to bang her."

"Yes," I whispered while my hands instinctively hovered around the binder clip, a primal urge building within me to remove the cruel device from my tortured clit. I knew I wouldn't be able to resist the temptation for long, and in that moment of vulnerability, I desperately cried out, “Please, hold my arms down! I can’t stop myself!”

“Fuck, it’s like she wants us to rape her,” Theo laughed, his eyes fixated on my writhing body as he and Bernard swiftly grabbed my arms, pulling them above my head. Their strong grip held me captive as if it were an extension of the paper clip’s own relentless torment.

The roughness of their touch only fueled the spasms surging through my body. The pain seemed to amplify my submission as if my entire existence was now at the mercy of these men who found perverse pleasure in my suffering. Yet, I was still determined not to use my safe word.

“Look at her tits shaking. It’s like... It follows her crying,” Albert remarked, his lustful gaze devouring the sight of my young tips bouncing on the rhythm of the contortions generated by the combination of Harvey’s relentless pounding, the binder clip’s merciless bite, and the men holding my arms above my head.

“Nothing better than a beautiful blonde bitch being fucked in the ass while she’s held down,” Charles added, his voice thick with desire and amusement. “She’s quite the show.”

My body trembled uncontrollably, every nerve ending on fire as the men continued to watch me with a mix of lust and delight. Their eyes feasted upon my naked form, taking in every shudder and convulsion that rippled through my flesh.

And I loved every second of it.

“Damn, just holding down a tight little blonde like her is hot enough,” Stanley commented. “But seeing her like this... all fucked up and helpless? It’s fucking erotic.”

“Her tears and that goddamn binder clip... it’s like a work of art,” Victor added, his voice dripping with carnal desire. “Just look at those pretty eyes welling up. She’s so fucking broken.”

As their crude words washed over me, I felt an odd mixture of shame and arousal. Something within me craved the debasement, the raw intensity of being used and degraded by these men who saw me as nothing more than a collection of holes to use, share, fill, and torment.

"About time a bitch's clit got some payback," Francis sneered, his eyes fixed on the cruel metal clamp between my legs. "Always having to service those needy things, licking and sucking them just to make our women happy. It feels good to see one get what it deserves."

"Fuck yeah," agreed Cliff, rubbing his crotch lewdly. "I could watch this all day, all week, just seeing her squirm and cry because of that useless clit. Feels good to be in control for once."

Their words echoed through my mind, reinforcing my position beneath them. My body, my pain, my humiliation—all of it was for their pleasure, and they reveled in it, which made me proud. I've always enjoyed pleasuring old men with my young body, and on that evening, on that tropical beach, 31 old cocks were vibrating because of what I had begged them to do me—to my clit. I was really the one in control!

"Such a perfect little fuck toy," Albert whispered, and I could hear his breath hitching with excitement. "Can't wait to have a turn with that tight ass of hers."

The men's crude laughter continuously filled the air, mingling with the sounds of my sobs, ragged gasps, screeches, and screams. It was a good thing we were on an isolated, small tropical island and that the resort staff had been notified to ignore anything happening with the naked gal.

"Damn," Charles muttered, his voice rough with arousal. "I've seen clit torture in porn before, but this is some next-level shit."

"Right?" agreed Stanley, his fingers digging into his bulging erection through his pants. "And it's even better because she's such a fucking hottie. Can't find someone as gorgeous as her in those videos."

My body suffering in front of them on that beach was more erotic to them than any porn video they had seen. Maybe I should consider a change of career.

"Bet those porn stars can't handle it as well as our little Delisha here," Edgar chimed in. "She's taking it like a champ, even though you can see that it hurts like hell. Damn! This is serious screeching!"

As they continued to discuss my predicament, I could feel my body responding to their rude words, a perverse thrill rushing through my veins as the reality of my submission excited me.

"Damn right," Albert agreed, the lust in his voice unmistakable. "You know, I would fuck a perfect babe like her anytime, anywhere! Whether my wife finds out or not. But her tears only make her more irresistible. God, I want my cock in her while she screams like that."

"And imagine... We have that fuck doll all week!"

This idea of torturing my clit to provide a better cock milking experience in my ass was my idea, but this was just the first cock to benefit from it. There were 30 other hard rods eagerly waiting around me on the beach. And they were already talking about doing it regularly all week.

As I kept howling and crying, I wondered if it had been such a good idea. I loved it, but will I still love it 31 times per day, all week?

Meanwhile, Harvey continued to pound into my ass relentlessly, each thrust causing the pain in my clit to intensify. I could barely breathe, overwhelmed by sobs, shrieks, and the raw sensation of being used like a cheap, dirty whore. Every single heartbeat sent surges of pain through me, making my butthole clench around Harvey's cock. I sure hope his cock, my god, was enjoying it. And he finally reassured me.

"Fuck, baby girl, your ass is so tight," Harvey groaned, clearly savoring his cock massage.

"Is she worth it?" Theo asked, smirking at Harvey while I remained pinned beneath him.

"Definitely," Harvey replied, his grip tightening on my hips as he drove himself deeper into my ass.

"Make her suffer more," another man suggested, his eyes filled with lustful hunger.

"God, yes..." I whispered, tears streaming down my cheeks. "Make my ass worship your cock."

Finally, Harvey reached his climax, grunting as he filled my butthole with his hot seed. He withdrew, panting, and looked down at me with a mixture of satisfaction and contempt. And he didn't immediately remove the binder clip. Instead, he reached over my quivering body and kissed me on the mouth.

"You're such a good sport, girl!" And then, as he cupped both of my young tits with his big hands, he added, "And so gorgeous!"

Eventually, he brought his attention back to my pussy. Grasping the binder clip, he unceremoniously removed it from my throbbing clit.

"Fuck!" I screamed, my body convulsing violently from the rush of blood flowing back into the sensitive flesh.

"Damn, did you see that?" Wilfred exclaimed, his eyes wide with excitement. "When Harvey removed the clip, her whole body shook like she was getting electrocuted. That could be an even better massage."

"Are you kidding me?" Theo chimed in, licking his lips in anticipation. "I'm gonna try that with my cock up her ass."

The second man in line didn't give me a break. Victor positioned himself between my legs. His thick cock pressed against my tight, young asshole, and I braced myself for another round of torment.

"Watch this," Victor said with a wicked grin as he shoved his cock deep into my ass, making me gasp in a mixture of pain and pleasure. He reached down, clamping the painful clip on my throbbing clit once more. My eyes widened as he snapped it off and then quickly put it back on, causing my entire body to jerk violently. The men around us laughed uproariously, relishing my suffering.

"Fuck, her ass is milking my cock like crazy!" Victor moaned, his thrusts growing more erratic.

He pounded into me mercilessly, his hips slamming against my ass cheeks. I whimpered and squirmed, overwhelmed by the sensations flooding my body—pain and pleasure, humiliation and ecstasy, all twisting together into a maelstrom of perverse delight.

Each thrust of that wrinkled old cock inside me, each bite of the clip on my ruined clit, brought me closer to the blissful oblivion I craved. My mind was blank, wiped clean of any thought beyond worshipping those cocks and the men who wielded them. They could do anything they wanted to me, and I would beg for more. I was put on this earth to pleasure them, to be used and tormented for their enjoyment.

"Keep doing it!" I begged through gritted teeth and screeches, tears streaming down my face. "Make it better for you!"

"Such a dirty little fuck toy," Charles commented.

Victor finished inside me, leaving my ass filled with his cum. Next, Albert stepped up, smirking as he pushed his cock into my abused hole. Just as Victor had done, he played with the binder clip on and off my clit, sending shockwaves of pain and ecstasy through me. The men continued to laugh at my misery.

"Please," I sobbed, "don't stop! It's what I'm here for."

Albert grunted in agreement, pounding away at my ass while torturing my swollen clit. By the time he finished, I was a trembling, tear-soaked mess after only three men.

The moment they snapped the tight metal clamp on my clit and the moment they took it off was the most painful. It was pure pain. And they were doing it repeatedly.

"Your turn, Stan," Albert announced, stepping away from my battered body.

Stanley took his place, driving his cock into my young asshole, and like the others, he toyed with the binder clip. The pain had become almost unbearable, but I couldn't deny the insane satisfaction at seeing the pleasure they were experiencing from my body's involuntary reactions.

I knew I wouldn't have it any other way. Since I started exploring my sexuality as a teenager, I believed my body was designed to pleasure old men. And that is what my body was being used for on that beach. I was where I belonged.

"Did you like it, bitch? On and off is better?" Theo asked, chuckling darkly.

"It hurts so much when you put it on and off," I cried, knowing it would excite them. "But do you like it? Does it make your cocks hard?"

"Well, fuck ya!" a chorus around me answered.

"It's all that matters!" I replied, between two screeching sessions. "My body is here for your cocks. Beat my clit! All of you. I want all of you!"

A few men simultaneously expressed surprise.

"All of us?"

"Yes... please... I need to worship more cocks."

"Greedy little whore, aren't you?" one man commented, stepping forward to take his turn.

"She's got the kind of tight young cunt that could make any sugar daddy go broke just to fuck her. And look at her golden hair and those perfect tits," another chimed in, his eyes devouring my body. "She could have any man she wants, but here she is, begging us old geezers to rape her ass."

My purpose, my reason for existing, was to bring these men joy through my suffering. The pain was a reward, proof of my devotion, and a path to transcendence.

"Please... don't stop," I whispered, my voice hoarse from crying out. "I want all cocks to use me like the cheap whore I am."

"Never thought I'd get to see such a perfect piece of ass willingly let herself be fucked so brutally," a man mused, rubbing his fingers against my lips.

"Hey!" shouted one of the men from the group of 17, looking over at the men from the group of 14. "How's this clit-torture milking compare to that footjob you had her do on the gravel?"

"Man, there's no comparison," replied one of my owners, grinning lasciviously. "This is so much tighter, and the way her butthole clenches when you pull that clip off... It's fucking amazing."

The sensations emanating through me as each man entered were unbearable yet unbearably pleasurable; my body stretched to impossible limits. Each time, adrenaline pulsed fiercely through me, like lightning along a wire, as each man fastened the paper clip around my bundle of nerves. The hard metal bit into my clitoris, pushing my pleasure to a dangerous level and sending me screeching and crying again. And then they would take it off, and the cycle of pain would continue.

"Her screams are music to my ears," an old man added, smirking cruelly as he watched my body convulse in pain. "Nothing's better than hearing a beautiful woman beg for more while we tear her apart."

I could see the twisted satisfaction in their eyes as they continued to use and abuse me. It was about more than just getting off; it was a power trip, a way for them to exert control over not only my body but also my mind. I knew deep down that their cruelty stemmed from past experiences with women who had made them feel weak or inadequate.

I was giving them a chance to claim their manhood back.

"Never thought I'd get revenge on all those stuck-up bitches who made me go down on them," one man grumbled, his grip tightening around my wrists as another man raped my ass. "But this... this is better than I ever imagined."

"Damn right," another agreed, smirking wickedly as he watched my helpless form squirm on the sand. "No more licking pussy like a good little boy; now we're in charge and making this hot piece of ass pay for them all."

"Hold her arms tight," the man inside of me yelled. "I'm gonna rape that bitch!"

I wasn't surprised by that statement. As the evening progressed, men were becoming more violent, and some of them clearly had a deep urge to vent anger against blondes, young women, all women —whatever it was, I was there to help them.

I was their therapist.

And despite the growing pain, the humiliation, and the sheer brutality of what was happening to me, something inside me refused to give up. I wanted to prove to them—and to myself—that I could take whatever they dished out, that I could be everything they desired and more.

I wanted to be the cure to emasculation, all while providing them with the best cock massage they ever had.

The pain and pleasure continued to blur together as men took turns savagely beating my ass, the binder clip snapping on and off my clit.

Cocks were my gods, and serving them was my purpose.

My mind grew hazy from the onslaught of sensations, and then... Fade to black! I passed out.

PHASE III

The Rest of The Week

19

A Soothing Embrace

Gently, I stirred from my slumber, feeling the soft sand beneath me. The salty sea breeze kissed my skin as the hypnotic sound of the waves crashing near my feet lulled me back to consciousness. In that moment, I reveled in the sensual embrace of the tropical paradise, nude on the beach with sand adhering to my silky flesh, my long blonde hair tangled and wild.

As my mind began to clear, flashes from the previous evening flooded back to me. My body had been used and abused by a group of ravenous old men taking turns to satisfy their primal desires. I remembered my ass being fucked relentlessly while they snapped a big metal binder paperclip onto my tender clit. They circled around me like hungry wolves, eager to feast upon my nubile form. The pain was indescribable yet intoxicating.

But wait a minute! There was a hand still on my body. Harvey! He was asleep next to me on the beach, in his t-shirt and bathing suit.

I tried to piece together the fragments of memory, eventually realizing that I must have passed out from the sheer intensity of it all. The thought excited me – I had finally found the limit of my tolerance to pain – but also left me disappointed. As their sex object, it was my duty to endure whatever torture they chose to inflict upon my clitoris. To pass out was to fail them, and that weighed heavily on my heart.

But now, waking up on this beautiful beach, I felt alive and connected to the world around me. The moonlight bathed my supple body, illuminating every curve and contour, casting an ethereal glow upon my delicate frame. My nude form was a living testament to the raw and carnal desires we had unleashed on the small island within the first 36 hours of our week-long dive trip.

Yet, my mind kept going back to last night. As I lay nude on the beach, the full weight of my failure settled upon me. I had passed out while they tortured me, betraying my purpose as their pain slut and denying them the satisfaction they craved. The sorrow gnawed at me, but I couldn't voice it with Harvey fast asleep by my side.

In the moonlight, I noticed my collar and leash discarded in the sand beside me. It assumed Harvey had removed them after I had lost consciousness. Now, I was completely nude – not a single piece of jewelry or clothing adorned my fragile form. I took a moment to examine my body, laid bare for all to see.

The soft glow of the moon highlighted the gentle curve of my breasts, their pert nipples hardened by the night's cool breeze. My long, slender legs stretched out before me, encased in a fine layer of damp sand that clung to my smooth skin like a second, gritty layer. My tiny, hairless mound was exposed, with the delicate folds of my labia slightly parted, revealing the tender pink flesh within. The waves lapped at my feet, sending tingles up my spine, a reminder of the primal force that surrounded me.

I shifted my gaze to my hands, resting on my taut belly, fingers splayed across the smooth expanse of flesh. The moon cast shadows between each digit, accentuating the vulnerability of my nakedness. The sight of my utterly exposed body filled me with a strange feeling of exhilaration, making my heart pound faster in my chest.

As I contemplated my situation, I couldn't help but admit to myself that, even in failure, there was an undeniable beauty in my raw, unadorned female form. Despite my disappointment, the eroticism of my nudity – the way my body seemed to meld with the sand and the ocean – stirred a strong sense of connection to the world around me.

I vowed then and there that I would do whatever it took to make up for my shortcomings. I would endure any pain, any humiliation, as long as it meant fulfilling my role as a plaything for those men who craved the pleasure that only my young, lithe woman body could provide.

In that moment, I made a silent promise to myself – and to them – that I would not falter again.

With a mixture of determination and trepidation, I sat up on the sand, my bare buttocks pressing against the gritty surface. The cool ocean breeze caressed my exposed body, making my nipples harden with a mix of arousal and chill. My eyes were drawn to the moonlit waves gently lapping at the shore, beckoning me toward their embrace.

My sudden movement seemed to stir Harvey from his slumber. He blinked groggily and gradually focused his gaze on me. Our eyes locked, and for a moment, time seemed to stand still. There was an undeniable eroticism in our shared silence as if the very air around us crackled with tension. I could feel his eyes tracing the contours of my nude female form, studying every inch of my delicate, vulnerable flesh.

"Delisha," he croaked, his voice hoarse with sleep. "How are you feeling?"

He moved closer to me, sitting down beside me on the sand. His concern seemed genuine, almost paternal, despite the fact I barely knew the old man. I stared at him, my mind struggling to reconcile this tender, caring man with the wild beast who had orchestrated my brutal abuse just hours before. It was disconcerting, but it also stirred something deep within me, a desire to understand the complexities that lay beneath men's often contradictory actions.

"Your clit..." he continued hesitantly, his gaze flicking briefly to the spot between my legs before returning to my face. "Is it okay?"

I remained silent, watching him intently. His concern puzzled me, but it also kindled a strange warmth in my chest, a feeling of connection that transcended our roles as tormentor and victim. Perhaps there was more to Harvey than I had initially thought, more than just a ringleader bent on inflicting pain and degradation upon my willing young female body.

As I pondered these thoughts, I couldn't help but feel a renewed sense of purpose, a determination to prove myself not only to him but to all the men in our traveling group who saw me as nothing more than a plaything for their twisted desires. I would embrace my role as their sex object with open arms, and I would endure whatever pain they inflicted upon me without complaint or hesitation.

After all, I had organized this dive trip with old men precisely to enjoy a full week of being a sex object.

Despite the peaceful surroundings, a jolt of pain brought me back to reality. Harvey's question about my clit made me hyper-aware of the searing agony emanating from that small, abused nub of flesh. I let out a strained laugh, realizing that my body had grown so accustomed to the near-constant torment inflicted upon it that my mind hadn't even registered the pain until he mentioned it.

"Really?" I managed to choke out, my voice laced with both amusement and a touch of self-mockery. The irony wasn't lost on me: my clit had been transformed from a source of pleasure into a tool for men to vent accumulated anger at clits they had been forced to lick or women who had disappointed them. And there I was, laughing at the absurdity of it all.

"Please, tell me what happened," I implored, meeting Harvey's gaze with a mixture of curiosity and determination. I needed to know the truth, no matter how brutal or humiliating it might be. My role as a sex object for these men demanded nothing less.

Harvey hesitated for a moment before explaining how I had passed out while one of the men fucked my ass and cruelly snapped the large metal paperclip onto my clit. As he recounted the events, something inside me stirred – a strange mixture of shame and pride that sent a shiver down my spine.

"I'm so sorry," I whispered, unable to tear my eyes away from his. "I failed all of you."

"It's not your fault, baby girl," Harvey assured me, attempting to assuage my guilt. "We pushed you too far."

"No," I insisted, shaking my head emphatically. "It's my job to serve and please you in whatever way you desire. I let you down, and I won't let it happen again."

My words were met with a solemn nod from Harvey, who seemed to understand the depth of my commitment to fulfilling my role as their personal sex slave and pain slut.

"Harvey, I want to resume the clit torture sessions as soon as the men are up," I said determinedly, my heart pounding in my chest at the thought of more degradation and pain.

"Delisha, first you need to check your clit," Harvey insisted, his voice gentle but firm. "Touch it and see how it feels."

With a reluctant sigh, I reached down and gingerly touched my throbbing clit. I winced at the sharp pain that shot through me, but stubbornly, I refused to back down.

"It hurts, but I can take it," I argued, my eyes locked with his. "I want them to continue abusing me. I need it."

"Delisha, you have to give your clit a break," Harvey implored, his eyes filled with concern. "We can still abuse the rest of your body, but we need to let that part of you heal."

"Only if you promise that you'll all continue treating me like a sex object for the rest of the week... non-human... a cock sleeve," I demanded, my resolve unwavering.

"Alright," Harvey finally agreed, his voice thick with reluctance. "I promise. We'll find other ways to use and abuse you without causing further harm to your clit."

"Deal," I whispered, a sense of satisfaction flooding through me. I had secured my place as their willing sex slave for the remainder of the week, just as I desired – the week wouldn't be a total failure.

And so, with our deal sealed, I prepared myself for the days ahead – days filled with debauchery, depravity, and the all-consuming desire to serve my Masters and Owners in any way they desired.

"Come on, Delisha. You should get some sleep in a bed," Harvey suggested, his voice heavy with exhaustion.

"No, I want to stay here on the beach," I replied, captivated by the beauty of the night and the cool sand beneath me. "I feel one with the ocean, the palm trees, and the sand. I'll be fine."

"But you need rest, Delisha. After all we've done to you..." he trailed off, concern etched across his face.

"Trust me, Old Man. I'll be okay," I insisted, my eyes locked onto his. He hesitated for a moment before reluctantly nodding and walking away, leaving me alone on the beach.

The moonlight danced on the water's surface as I stood up, feeling an irresistible pull towards the ocean. My naked body embraced the breeze, unburdened by clothing or inhibition. With each step, my feet sunk into the cool, wet sand, heightening my connection to this natural paradise.

As I walked into the gentle waves, I felt their soothing caress against my swollen labia and tortured clit. A delicious shiver ran through me, contrasting the pain from earlier abuse with the tender touch of the ocean. I stopped, allowing the waves to repeatedly wash over my vulnerable pussy, bringing a strange sense of comfort and pleasure.

Submerged in the rhythmic embrace of the sea, I reveled in my nakedness, in the purest form of communion with nature. And though my body ached from the torment it had endured, I felt alive, powerful, and so beautifully connected to the world around me.

Feeling the ocean's loving embrace around my tender clit, I continued to wade deeper into the water. The waves gradually grew higher, soon reaching my flat, seductive belly. A mixture of exhilaration and vulnerability washed over me as the cool water caressed my smooth skin, heightening my senses. I closed my eyes for a moment, allowing myself to feel truly connected to the natural world around me.

As I ventured further, the waves began to lap at my young, erotic breasts. The sensation of the water teasing my nipples sent shivers through my body, not from the cold but from the sheer excitement of it all. I stopped, allowing the rhythmic motion of the waves to gently massage my sensitive breasts, giving in to their hypnotic touch.

The group of old men had made me their dive gear slave and denied me the pleasure of scuba diving. But I didn't need a regulator in my mouth to feel one with the ocean.

The buoyancy of my full, perky breasts made them float atop the water, bobbing up and down with each wave. The sight of my own floating breasts, bathed in moonlight, stirred something primal within me. I felt like an enchanting siren of the sea, my body an irresistible lure to any man who dared to gaze upon it.

"Is this what it means to be an erotic creature?" I wondered to myself. As I stood there, naked and vulnerable, my body fully exposed to the elements, I was intoxicated by the realization that I was more than just an object for men's pleasure. In this wild, natural, tropical environment, I was also a powerful force of nature, able to wield my sexuality on my terms.

Lost in the intimate dance between my body and the ocean, I reveled in the knowledge that despite the degradation and abuse I had willingly endured, I still possessed the power to define my desires. Embracing the contradictions that lay at the heart of my carnal appetites, I felt a newfound sense of freedom and strength surge through me.

"Let them worship me," I thought, a wicked grin spreading across my face. "For I am both their willing victim and their untamed goddess."

Finally, I couldn't resist the allure of the ocean any longer. I dove in and began to swim, my youthful buttocks round and supple as they emerged at the surface with each stroke. The cool water felt refreshing against my naked skin, and I reveled in the sensation of weightlessness that enveloped me.

I swam back toward the shore, intoxicated by the beauty of my surroundings and the feeling of complete freedom that came from being naked in the embrace of the sea. In shallow water near the shore, I sat down on the underwater sand, my thighs parted slightly as the waves continued to gently caress my body.

The rhythmic motion of the water caused the sand beneath me to shift and swirl, massaging my tender pussy with each passing wave. The sensation was electrifying, sending jolts of pleasure through my core as the granules brushed against my sensitive, swollen clit – a reminder of the brutal treatment it had endured earlier.

As wave after wave washed over me, I could feel my breasts being cradled by the gentle current, their buoyancy causing them again to lift and lower in the water. It was as if the ocean itself was teasing and tantalizing my body, stoking the fires of my desire even further.

"Is this what paradise feels like?" I mused to myself, my mind awash with sensations and emotions that were both thrilling and overwhelming. In that moment, I felt a profound connection to the world around me - to the vast expanse of the ocean, to the moonlit sky above, and to the primal forces that governed the tides and the seasons.

"Let them try to tame me," I thought defiantly, my heart swelling with pride. "For as long as I have the ocean by my side, I will always be free." And with that thought, I surrendered myself completely to the waves, allowing them to wash away any lingering doubts or fears and leaving behind only the pure, untainted essence of who I truly was – a wild, untamed goddess of the sea.

20

A Dirty Girl

I awoke to the gentle lapping of waves at my feet, the swaying palm trees above creating a natural symphony as the wind rustled through their leaves. There I was, completely nude, with no clothes or jewelry in sight, lying on warm tropical sand and truly one with nature. The feeling was intoxicating, like paradise itself had wrapped me in its embrace.

As I lay there, basking in the sensual freedom of my nudity, I began to explore my body with my fingertips. The sand had mixed with the salt from the ocean to leave a sticky, gritty texture on my skin, adding a raw, primal element to my touch. I trailed my fingers along the curves of my breasts, down my abdomen, and over the delicate folds between my thighs, relishing in the sensation of being so dirty and exposed.

The smell of saltwater and sweat clung to me like a lover's embrace, a heady reminder of my innate connection to the elements. I reveled in this newfound filthiness, feeling more alive and erotic than ever before.

As I caressed my skin, reveling in the way every part of my body was coated in sand and dried saltwater, a wicked thought danced through my mind: men loved calling me a dirty girl as they took pleasure in my body. But now, I was quite literally dirty, an untamed creature of the sea and sand. The idea thrilled me, and I longed for a group of men to bear witness to my wild, uninhibited state.

My laughter bubbled up within me, echoing my thoughts, as I imagined those men devouring me with their eyes, worshipping my exposed form with an almost religious fervor. I knew that, as a sex object meant for their pleasure, I should feel degraded or ashamed – but instead, I felt empowered and excited by the prospect of surrendering myself to their desires.

As I rose from the golden sands, I caught a glimpse of my tiny, young body, every curve and contour on full display for anyone who might happen upon this beach. Sand clung to my skin in various places, accentuating the roundness of my breasts and the inviting swell of my hips. My hair, long and blonde, was tangled with sand and salt crystals that glistened in the early morning light.

Feeling the urge to cleanse my body, I rose and made my way toward the ocean. The waves called to me like a siren's song, drawing me into their cool embrace. As I entered the water, I felt it wrap around me, soothing my battered body.

Submerging myself beneath the surface, I began to run my hands over my skin, letting the saltwater work its magic on my sand-coated body. I moved my fingers in slow, deliberate strokes, relishing in the sensation of cleansing myself of the grime that clung to me. My hands delicately traced the contours of my breasts, gliding down my abdomen and along my thighs as I washed away the remnants of my sandy bed.

I dipped my head under the surface, allowing the water to envelop my hair. I gathered my long, blonde locks in my hands and gently squeezed, watching as the salty water flowed through them, carrying away the dirt and sand. The intimate act of washing my hair felt almost sinful as if I were indulging in some forbidden pleasure.

As I emerged from the ocean, I was struck by a thought that sent a wicked smirk across my face. If I continued to sleep outdoors, salt would stick to my body again and again as it dried after each swim. My hair would remain a tangled mess, lacking the tools to tame it. The idea of being such a dirty girl for the rest of the trip excited me beyond measure. After all, blondes and dirty girls have more fun, and I was both.

My heart raced with anticipation as I envisioned the reactions of the men in our group, their lustful gazes fueled by my unkempt appearance. I knew that I was playing into their fantasies, willingly offering myself up as a filthy, erotic creature for their enjoyment – and I couldn't wait for every deliciously debauched moment yet to come.

The sun had already risen by the time I began walking toward the resort's main building, my wet hair trailing down my back and my nude body glistening from the seawater. As I approached, I noticed most of the men were on the dock, preparing for the morning boat dive. I realized I had missed breakfast, but it didn't bother me. I was committed to only consuming male semen all week, which I lovingly referred to as "male milk." The taste and texture of semen were divine to me, and I knew there would be plenty available on the dive boat.

As I neared the dock, every eye turned toward me, taking in my nakedness. I felt dirty, the dried salt clinging to my skin and my hair a wild, tangled mess. The sensation thrilled me. I entertained myself with the image of being a filthy outdoor nude animal, approaching my owners on the dock to be petted. The thought sent shivers of excitement through my body as I reveled in the role of submissive sex pet.

My footsteps grew more confident, my hips swaying seductively while I walked toward the group of old men who eagerly observed my approach. Their gazes traced every curve and dip of my body, lingering on my breasts and between my legs. I could feel their hunger for me, their carnal desires simmering just below the surface.

As I finally reached my Owners, the men's eyes seemed to bore into my flesh, taking in every inch of my exposed form. My nipples hardened under their scrutiny, betraying my arousal at being so brazenly displayed. And as I stood there, basking in their lustful attention and feeling like a dirty, erotic creature, I knew that I was truly in my element and wouldn't have it any other way.

"About time you showed up," Harvey barked, his hand coming down on my ass with a stinging slap. "Now get to work setting up the gear for all of us."

"Yes, Sir," I replied, eager to fulfill my role as their dive gear slave for the week. The sharp sting in my buttocks only served to heighten my arousal, reminding me of my submissive position.

I moved to the storage area and began carrying each man's dive gear onto the boat, one by one. As I bent over to pick up the heavy equipment, I could feel their lustful eyes following the curve of my bare backside, taking in every exposed inch of me. With each step, I felt the weight of their gazes and the cool sea breeze brushing my naked skin.

My nipples hardened beneath their stares, betraying my excitement at being so totally nude. The sensation of being vulnerable in front of these men sent a rush through me, fueling the fire that smoldered deep inside. As I carried each set of gear, the men would occasionally reach out to slap or grope my ass, further asserting their dominance over me and reinforcing my status as their plaything.

As I worked, I reveled in the feeling of being both a sex slave and a dive gear slave – a nude one. It was a deliciously erotic combination that made my body hum with anticipation. I love scuba diving as much as I love being a sex pet. Therefore, the thought of spending the entire week like this, submitting to their every whim, filled me with an intoxicating mixture of fear and desire. Their rough hands caressing, grabbing, and slapping my exposed flesh sent shivers coursing through me, and I loved every second of it.

Each time I completed a task, I'd look up to see their hungry eyes devouring me, satisfied with my obedience but craving more. And with every touch, every whispered command, every demeaning comment, I felt more and more like a piece of meat presented for their pleasure. But instead of feeling degraded or ashamed, I embraced this role with open arms.

As the boat pulled away from the dock, I moved from one set of dive gear to the next, diligently preparing each piece for the 14 men – my Owners – who watched me intently. They lounged around the boat, their gazes never straying far from my naked female form as I worked. The salty ocean breeze teased my skin, making my nipples harden under their lecherous stares. It thrilled me to be the center of their attention, the sole focus of their lust.

"Hey Delisha," one of the men, Fred, called out. "How's your clit today? Looks like we really did a number on you last night."

I hesitated for a moment, feeling a twinge of pain at the reminder of the previous night's events. "It hurts quite a bit," I admitted, my cheeks flushing with embarrassment. "I'm sorry I passed out while you were playing with me."

"Ah, don't worry about it," Harvey chimed in, his voice authoritative yet reassuring. "We can still have our fun with you; we'll just give your clit a break to heal up."

I remained silent. While part of me was glad for the temporary reprieve from the torment, another part craved the rough handling and degradation that came with it.

As I resumed setting up the dive gear, I could feel the eyes of the men following my every move, studying the curve of my ass, the bounce of my young breasts, and the sway of my hips. Even though they couldn't touch my most sensitive spot, I knew they were still fantasizing about the many other ways they could use and abuse me throughout the week. And the thought sent a shiver of anticipation through my body.

Their conversations grew more animated, punctuated by laughter and crude jokes about my body and the things they wanted to do to me. It was as if they were trying to outdo each other in their lewdness, and I reveled in the raw, unfiltered desire that poured from their mouths.

"Hey, Delisha," Theo called out suddenly, his tone teasing but also slightly concerned. "You sure you're okay with us still having our fun with you, even though your clit's off-limits for now?"

I paused in my work, looking up at him with a mischievous smile. "Yes, Sir," I responded, my voice dripping with eagerness. "I'm here to serve you and satisfy your desires, remember? So go ahead, use me however you want. But please don't forget to feed me!"

The men exchanged excited glances, and I could see the predatory gleam in their eyes as they took in my words.

Feeling the curious stares of the men, I knew they wanted a closer look at the source of my pain and vulnerability. Their fascination with my clit was both humiliating and thrilling, and I decided to indulge them. Climbing onto a bench in the middle of the boat, I positioned myself so that my intimate area was at eye level for the men.

"Alright, gentlemen," I said, trying to sound confident despite my exposed state. "Here it is."

I spread my outer vaginal lips and pushed the hood up, revealing my swollen, tender clitoris. The men leaned in, taking in every detail of the small, sensitive piece of flesh that had brought me so much agony the night before.

"Can't believe that tiny thing made you pass out," one man snickered, his eyes locked on my clit.

"Imagine being such a defective fuck doll that your own body betrays you," another chimed in, laughing cruelly.

Their comments stung, but I couldn't deny the twisted thrill it gave me, knowing these men saw me as nothing more than their toy. As they continued to make derogatory remarks about my clitoris, I kept it exposed, allowing them to openly mock and degrade me.

"Who'd want to waste their time pleasuring that?" one man scoffed. "It's barely even visible!"

"Seriously, why do women even have those things?" someone else grumbled. "Just stick to sucking our cocks, and we'll all be happier."

The men laughed heartily while I stood there, still holding my lips apart, feeling like a piece of meat on display. But deep down, I loved it – the raw, unfiltered desires of these old men, the way they objectified and dehumanized me. It was all so intoxicating, and I couldn't get enough of it.

"Alright, sweetie," one of the men called out, grinning wickedly. "Since you're such a pro at entertaining us, how about giving us some dirty jokes about that little clit of yours?"

"Sure thing, boys," I obliged, still holding my lips open and exposing my clit for their amusement. I had to admit, I loved making them laugh, even if it meant poking fun at myself and other young women like me.

"What do blondes and clitorises have in common? They both love attention but can be hard to find when needed!"

The men chuckled and nudged each other, urging me to continue. I racked my brain for more crude jokes, feeling a bizarre sense of pride in being able to entertain these old men with my body and humor.

"Alright, let's see... What's the difference between a clitoris and a golf ball?" I paused for dramatic effect, my fingers still gripping my lips apart to keep my clit exposed. "Men will actually look for a golf ball!"

The men roared with laughter, and I felt a surge of satisfaction at having made them happy, even if it meant mocking my own kind.

"Keep 'em coming, girl!" one man shouted, egging me on.

Their laughter filled the boat, and as I stood there naked on the bench, holding my vaginal lips open and clit exposed just to entertain this group of old men, I truly felt like a piece of meat. But I loved it. There was something incredibly exhilarating about being seen as a non-human piece of flesh to be devoured by these perverted men – it fed into my darkest desires and fueled my lust for submission.

"Alright, last one! Why do men get lost in the female genitalia? Because even the clitoris comes with a hood!" The men laughed uproariously once more, and I couldn't help but feel a sense of accomplishment.

As the laughter died down and the boat continued toward our dive site, I knew that my time aboard with these men would be filled with all manner of debauchery and degradation. But deep down, I also knew that there was nothing I craved more – to be seen as a sex object, a piece of meat for these old men to use and abuse as they saw fit. And in this twisted world of mine, that was pure bliss.

21

A Salty Surface Interval

As I stood on the boat, completely exposed in my nudity, I couldn't help but feel a twinge of excitement at the contrast between my tiny, vulnerable female body and the 14 old men surrounding me, all dressed in t-shirts and bathing suits. Their eyes roamed over my body, taking in every inch of my smooth, sun-kissed skin, the swell of my ample breasts, and the delicate curve of my hips. The boat captain and the dive resort divemaster, both clad in their own uniforms, expertly took care of their duties, but their gazes lingered on me as well. I reveled in the attention, savoring the way my bare flesh seemed to awaken a primal hunger within these men.

The boat arrived at the first dive site, and the divemaster quickly attached the boat to the mooring. I approached Ralph, our group's divemaster, feeling the cool ocean breeze caress my naked form. "You know, when we organized this trip, I was supposed to be diving with everyone," I began, a note of playful accusation in my voice. "But since these guys turned me into their sex slave and won't let me dive as punishment for being a cock tease, I hope you'll make sure they have a good time underwater and do it safely."

Ralph looked into my eyes, his gaze flicking down briefly to take in my nakedness before returning to my face. "Of course, Delisha," he replied, a hint of admiration in his voice. "I'll do my best to make sure everything goes smoothly while they're diving."

"Thank you," I said, smiling warmly at him. Though I loved my role as the group's submissive plaything, I also cared deeply about their safety and the success of the dive trip. With Ralph's assurance, I felt a little more at ease, knowing that someone would be keeping an eye on the men while they explored the depths of the ocean.

As Ralph and I continued our conversation, he pointed out how lucky he was to be on this trip. He had scored the free spot often offered by dive resorts to trip leaders. With a mischievous grin, he mentioned that everyone at the dive shop up North would kill to see me naked, though many had already seen me in various states of undress, of course.

Even though hundreds of men had seen me in the nude so far in my life, I couldn't help but feel a thrill at the thought of men wanting to see my naked body. I told Ralph that I'd make sure to stop by the dive shop when I went back up north to visit my parents. In response, he joked that they could organize a special evening with all the staff for me to do a striptease. It may have been a joke, but I loved the idea, envisioning their hungry eyes devouring my every move as I danced for them.

Meanwhile, the 14 men on the boat were busy putting on their dive gear and getting ready for the dive, completely ignoring me. It was only the second day of our week-long dive trip, and it seemed like they had already grown used to having my naked body around. Yesterday, they had tied me down during the dive, forcing me to stay aboard the boat and miss the experience. Today, they simply went about their business, leaving me feeling sad and almost invisible. Tears threatened to spill from my eyes at any moment.

On top of that, my love for the ocean called to me, making me want to grab a scuba kit and join the men below the waves. But wait! No! I didn't want to go diving; I wanted to be their sex slave, tied down and waiting for their return. The conflicting desires left me feeling utterly confused, my heart heavy with uncertainty.

As the men geared up and prepared to dive, I stood there naked, struggling with my emotions. I tried to focus on the warm sun and the gentle sway of the boat, but my thoughts kept returning to my role as a sex slave and my desire to dive beneath the surface. What would the rest of this trip hold for me? Would I find a way to reconcile these conflicting desires?

My heart sank when Harvey approached, noticing my sad expression. "What's wrong, Delisha?" he asked, genuine concern in his voice.

"Harvey, you promised that the men would keep abusing me even if my clit needed a break," I replied, my frustration evident. He nodded, remembering his words. "So why am I standing here free as a bird? If they were really abusing me, I wouldn't be able to just grab a scuba kit and dive with them."

Understanding dawned on Harvey's face, and he quickly took action. "Captain, can I have some rope?" he called out before turning back to me. "Get on your knees next to the bench," he ordered as the boat captain handed over the requested ropes.

As I obeyed, the men suddenly came to life around me, whistling and catcalling as they encouraged Harvey. "Yeah, tie her down, Harvey!" one shouted, while another added, "Make sure she stays put for us!"

"Keep her legs spread, too! We want a show!" someone else chimed in, drawing laughter from the crowd. Their crude comments and enthusiasm fueled my own desires, awakening the need within me to be utterly used and controlled.

Harvey knelt down beside me, wrapping the rope securely around my ankles and tying me to the bench. The knots were tight and unyielding, ensuring that I couldn't escape or move much at all. My legs were forced apart, leaving me completely exposed and vulnerable.

"Make sure she knows her place!" yelled an old man, leering at my helpless form.

"Can't wait to see our little lamb all tied up and ready to be slaughtered when we get back from the dive!" added another one, licking his lips hungrily.

As Harvey finished tying my ankles to the bench, he moved on to securing my wrists. He grabbed my arms and pulled them behind my back, wrapping another rope around my wrists and ensuring they were tightly bound together. I felt a shiver of anticipation run through me as I realized that there would be no escaping this position. Finally!

"Be ready to clean the ocean salt off our balls, cocks, and buttholes when we come back from the dive," Harvey growled in my ear, his breath hot against my skin. I couldn't help but feel a twinge of excitement at the prospect.

"But I'm hungry," I protested, looking up at him with pleading eyes.

Harvey considered me for a moment before smirking. "Maybe we'll let you eat our semen if you obey," he said, the crude suggestion sending another jolt of arousal through me.

"Thank you, Daddy," I whispered, feeling a mix of gratitude and humiliation at the thought of being reduced to such a base act just to satisfy my hunger.

The group of old men, now fully geared up for the dive, began to make their way off the boat. I watched them intently, a strange mixture of envy and pleasure coursing through me. On one hand, I longed to join them in exploring the underwater world I loved so dearly. But on the other hand, there was something undeniably thrilling about giving up that passion to serve as their submissive plaything – a cock tease in need of a lesson.

As the boat captain and divemaster focused on monitoring the divers' progress, I found myself alone with my thoughts. I couldn't help but relish the pain I felt – both physical and emotional – because it meant I was truly serving my purpose as a sex object.

Although my heart ached at the thought of missing out on the dive, it also swelled with pride, knowing I had willingly sacrificed my greatest love to satisfy these men's desires.

The conflicting emotions consumed me, but ultimately, my need for degradation and submission won out. And despite the ache in my chest, I knew this was where I belonged – as their willing sex slave, ready to be used and abused at their whim.

AS THE SCUBA divers began to resurface and return to the boat, they were greeted by the sight of my naked body, still bound and on display for their lewd enjoyment. The murmur of impressed voices and lustful chuckles filled the air as they climbed back aboard, unable to take their eyes off me.

"Damn, look at that girl's perfect tits," one man remarked, his gaze lingering on my chest.

"Her ass is just begging for a spanking," another chimed in, smirking at the thought.

"God, I could stare at her all day," a third admitted, clearly entranced by my bound form.

I felt a surge of heat and arousal course through me, knowing that I was the center of their attention, their raw desires focused entirely on my total nudity. I was sure that the way my wrists were tied behind me only heightened their perception of me as a piece of meat.

Despite their crude comments and barking laughter, none of the men made a move toward me until Harvey took charge. Dropping his bathing suit in front of my mouth, he ordered me to clean the salt from his balls and cock. With my hands still tied, I had no choice but to use my mouth to pleasure him.

Taking his heavy sack into my mouth, I swirled my tongue around each testicle, expertly removing every trace of salty ocean water. My lips then wrapped around his thick shaft, gliding up and down as I licked the length of his member with fervor. The taste of his skin mingled with the saltiness, creating an intoxicating blend that drove me wild.

"Oh, baby girl, you're such a talented little cocksucker," Harvey praised, grinning down at me as I worked my oral magic on him. My lack of hand movement seemed to only enhance the eroticism of the scene, proving that I was indeed an expert at pleasing men with just my mouth.

Soon, pubic hair from Harvey's crotch was trapped in my mouth, and I reveled in the discomfort. It was a reminder of my purpose – to be nothing more than an object for these men to use and enjoy. The coarse hairs tickled my tongue and caught between my teeth, making me want to gag, but I resisted.

"Look at our little slut, struggling with just a few hairs," Harvey teased, smirking down at me. "You should be grateful for every gift we give you, whore."

I tried to spit out the hairs, but he noticed and slapped me hard across the face. "Don't you dare reject your gifts, girl. It's impolite."

My cheeks flushed with shame, and I nodded, accepting my role. But Harvey seemed to understand that swallowing too much pubic hair could be unhealthy. He asked another man in the group to bring a glass of water while I continued to work on his cock.

Harvey held the glass to my lips, allowing me to rinse my mouth and spit out the water, along with the unwanted hairs. My hands were still tied behind my back, so I had no control over the process. With the water dribbling down my chin, Harvey slapped me again.

"Be a good slave, and don't reject your gifts," he scolded. Then, without missing a beat, he pushed his engorged cock back into my eager mouth.

At that moment, I think I was in love with Harvey. He was caring, finding a way to remove pubic hair from my mouth. Yet, at the same time, he punished me for it. Why can't all men be like him?

I sucked on him with renewed vigor, knowing that he both cared for my well-being and demanded total submission. I felt humbled and aroused by his treatment, embracing my role as a sex object even more.

Soon after, I felt the overwhelming sensation of Harvey's cock throbbing in my mouth, signaling his imminent release. With my hands still tied behind my back, I focused on using my tongue and lips to bring him to the edge. My blue eyes met his, allowing me to absorb every ounce of his domination over me. I swirled my tongue around the head of his cock, teasing him while maintaining eye contact.

"God, you're such a good little cocksucker," Harvey panted as he gripped my hair tightly.

Finally, he couldn't hold back any longer, and his hot semen filled my mouth. I eagerly accepted it, letting the warm, salty fluid coat my tongue. Harvey pulled his cock out and slapped my face, leaving a stinging sensation that made me feel even more submissive.

"Swallow everything, you filthy slut," he commanded, his voice dripping with authority and lust.

I obeyed without hesitation, swallowing every drop of his cum. I knew my purpose was to be a used and abused sex object, and I reveled in it. As I swallowed the last remnants of Harvey's essence, I looked up at him, eager for what would come next.

"Alright, boys, who's next?" Harvey called out to the other men. "That... thing... here is there to clean the salt off your balls. Don't be shy."

One man jumped forward and quickly dropped his bathing suit, exposing his hairy balls. "Get to work, slut," he said, pushing them towards my face.

Some other men chimed in, yelling obscenities about their salty buttholes also needing attention. The man in front of me turned around, presenting his hairy butthole for me to clean. Taking a deep breath, I leaned forward, my tongue darting out to lick the coarse hairs surrounding his puckered hole. As revolting as it was, I found myself oddly turned on by the debasement of it all.

"Look at the dumb blonde go," one man chuckled as I continued to lick and clean the man's hairy butthole. My face flushed with humiliation, but my body responded in a primal way, craving more degradation and abuse.

From an early age, I thought I was put on earth to be a sex slave, to be used and abused by men, especially old men. Why else was I given a body that made all cocks get so easily and naturally hard? Their harsh words and rough treatment only served as a reminder of my place in society – a reminder that I craved and needed.

I REMAINED ON MY KNEES, my wrists still tied behind my back, as the men took turns using the salt-cleaning device. The salty ocean air mixed with the scent of sweat and arousal, creating an atmosphere both intoxicating and erotic. Each man approached with his specific desires, and I was eager to fulfill them all.

"Wow, Delisha, you're a sight for sore eyes," one man commented as he admired my naked body, perfectly displayed for their viewing pleasure. The lust in his eyes made my heart race with excitement.

"Alright, who's next?" Harvey regularly called out, maintaining his position as the ring leader. One after another, the men presented themselves to me, their balls, cocks, and buttholes covered in salt from the ocean. I dutifully licked each of them clean, savoring the taste of their masculinity and submission.

"Look at you, you little slut," one old man rasped, standing in front of my mouth. He grasped a handful of my hair and yanked my head back, exposing my throat. "The only diving you'll be doing today is diving for balls."

Laughter erupted around me, and my already-soaked pussy clenched in response. Yes. This was my purpose, my reason for being.

"Here, let me help you rinse your mouth," a nice man said. With my hands tied, I was entirely reliant on him to lift the glass to my lips. I swished the water around in my mouth, the pubic hairs sticking to my tongue finally loosening. And then he pulled the glass away, making me spit the water out onto the boat floor.

As each man ejaculated into my eagerly waiting mouth, I relished in the feeling of being a true cum bucket. With every salty, warm load that filled my mouth, I felt more and more like the sex slave I was meant to be.

The crude sexual jokes and demeaning comments only fueled my desire to submit to their every whim. Their words, though harsh, served as a constant reminder of my place in society.

As the boat rocked gently on the waves, I continued to worship their salty cocks, balls, and buttholes like the sex object I was, knowing that this was where I truly belonged.

~

I DIDN'T MANAGE to service all fourteen men during the surface interval. I waited on my knees, tied, while they did their second dive of the morning. The sun beat down on my exposed body as I awaited their return, anticipating the tasks that lay ahead.

"Looks like we left some unfinished business here," one of the men remarked as they began to climb back onto the boat, dripping wet in their scuba gear. My naked body, wrists tied behind my back and vulnerable, seemed to be a captivating sight for these old men. I felt the heat between my legs increase as their eyes roamed over every inch of me.

"Baby girl, don't worry. We'll make sure you get your fill before we head back to shore," Harvey said with a wicked grin. I knew he understood my dark desires, and his words ignited a burning need within me to submit and continue my purpose as their sex object and cum bucket.

As the boat made its way back to shore, I resumed my role, licking salt off balls and buttholes, and sucking cocks with fervor. The men relished in my submission, groaning with pleasure and exchanging crude jokes about my willingness to degrade myself for their satisfaction.

"Can you believe how thirsty this little slut is for our old cocks?" one man laughed, grabbing a handful of my blonde hair as I sucked him off.

"Her mouth must be heaven for cocks," another chimed in, stroking himself while waiting his turn.

"Damn right," Harvey agreed, watching the scene unfold with a satisfied smirk.

By the time we reached the shore, I had taken fifteen loads of hot, sticky semen in my mouth, swallowing it all down hungrily. Harvey had returned for a second time, demanding I lick his butthole clean. I obliged, of course.

"Good girl," Harvey praised me, panting and sweaty from the experience. "You truly the best cocksucker and cum bucket."

"Thank you, Sir," I replied, my voice hoarse but filled with gratitude. As the boat docked, I knew that I had fully embraced my purpose.

Under the amused look of men on the dock, Harvey untied me so that I could start my second job – dive gear slave, in the nude, of course! I worked long hours during that dive trip; I can tell you that much!

22

The Afternoon Shift

The warm Caribbean breeze caressed my naked body as I walked towards the resort's restaurant. My head still buzzed from the morning of servicing my Owners, their semen providing sustenance for my hungry body. I was late to lunch, having finished rinsing and hanging the dive gear for the 14 men in my group. As I approached the outdoor dining area, my heart raced in anticipation of what awaited me.

Just before entering, I locked eyes with the general manager of the resort, a man who had known me since I was a young girl learning to scuba dive. We shared a tense moment of understanding, though no words were spoken. Our gazes held, acknowledging the unspoken agreement that allowed me to roam the resort as a wild, naked animal, fulfilling my Owners' every desire.

"Delisha," he began, his voice stern yet curious. "I heard about someone passing out on the beach last night. Care to explain? Guests passing out is not good for business."

I hesitated, my thoughts racing through the events of the previous evening – the paperclip tormenting my clit until I lost consciousness. "Well, you see," I said, a sultry smile spreading across my lips, "I'm not a guest here, am I? I didn't pay, don't eat the food, and don't even have a room. I'm more like a wild, nude animal roaming the resort."

The GM shook his head, clearly not impressed by my response. Yet, he turned and walked away, leaving me to enjoy my nudity and sexual activities.

Stepping into the restaurant area, I was instantly met with a barrage of whistles and catcalls from the men. They were already eating, their lustful eyes following my every move. I stood before them, uncertain of what to do since I had committed to consuming nothing but semen for the entire week. As they stared at me, I felt a rush of excitement and decided to take matters into my own hands.

With a sensual sway of my hips, I climbed onto one of the tables, positioning myself as the centerpiece for their enjoyment. Kneeling on the table, I spread my legs wide to expose my smooth, waxed pussy. Arching my back, my perky breasts thrust forward, demanding their attention. Lowering my eyes demurely, I placed my hands palm-up on my thighs, assuming the ultimate submissive position.

As lunch progressed, some of the men finished eating and began to approach me, examining my body like a precious piece of art. Harvey, the ringleader of my Owners, whistled loudly, demanding everyone's attention. "Gentlemen," he announced, "as we all know, our lovely Delisha here passed out last night due to some intense clit torture. So, her clit is off-limits while it heals. However, she remains the sex pet of this resort."

The room filled with murmurs and chuckles from the men, crude jokes about my blonde hair and young body echoing throughout the space. Their words only fueled my desire to be used and to worship the cocks of these old men.

The group of 17 old men had heard tales of my role as not just a sex pet but also a dive gear slave. Their eyes bore into me. "Think we could borrow the blonde for the afternoon?"

The group of 14, my Owners, discussed amongst themselves,

eventually agreeing to lend me to the other group for the afternoon. "But you must feed her your semen," Harvey insisted, smirking devilishly. "She needs it to survive, after all."

"Sure," the spokesman for the group of 17 agreed, eyeing me hungrily. "Now, go prepare our dive gear, girl."

I nodded obediently, standing up from my submissive position on the table and walking back to the dock, completely nude. My bare feet slapped against the sun-warmed wood, and the salty ocean breeze tickled my naked skin.

At the dive shop, I asked the staff which gear belonged to the group of 17, and they pointed me in the right direction. One by one, I carried the scuba kits onto the dive boat, my breasts swaying with each step and my tight ass jiggling enticingly. The weight of the gear was nothing compared to the overwhelming desire I felt to be used and abused by these men, to have their hot, sticky cum fill my mouth and nourish me.

As I finished loading the gear, I couldn't help but wonder what new experiences these 17 old men would bring, how they would use me in ways that would push my limits and make me feel like the perfect sex object I longed to be. My body ached with anticipation, and I knew that this afternoon would be one that I'd never forget.

WITH ALL THE dive gear loaded onto the boat, I stood on the deck, naked and vulnerable, as the 17 old men approached. My body was a buffet of delight for their hungry eyes. The group of 17 seemed even more eager to devour me than the group of 14 who owned me.

The captain and divemaster untied the boat, setting us on our way to the dive site. As soon as the engine roared to life, two men from the ravenous pack positioned themselves on either side of me. They didn't speak to me, treating me like the fuck doll I was. One man grabbed my hips, forcing me to bend over as he lined up his throbbing cock with my tight butthole. The other man grasped my head, guiding his engorged member into my waiting mouth.

As they spit-roasted me, I focused on the sensations coursing through my body. The way the man behind me gripped my hips tightly enough to leave bruises, the rough thrusts filling my ass, and the relentless pounding in my mouth as the other man rammed his cock down my throat. It was degrading, but it fueled the fire burning within me.

Throughout the journey to the dive site, the men took turns using my body for their pleasure. There was always one cock buried in my wet pussy or tight ass, and another filling my mouth. I could feel the power these old cocks held over me, and I worshipped them like the gods they were. Each time one of them was about to reach climax, they made sure to deposit their hot seed into my eager mouth, feeding me the semen I craved so much.

My body ached with each thrust and slap, but it was the pain I needed, the pain that made me feel alive. The taste of their cum in my mouth was a reminder of my purpose – to be used, to be consumed, to fulfill their every desire.

~

THE DIVE BOAT came to a stop at the dive site, its engine humming softly as the men eagerly prepared themselves for their underwater adventure. I watched them from a distance, my body still slick and glistening with sweat and semen, feeling like a discarded toy left behind once the novelty wore off. Their excitement was palpable, but I wasn't part of it. I was just an object to be used – and though that thought sent a shiver down my spine, I couldn't help but feel a pang of longing.

I had always loved the ocean, its vastness and depth calling out to the wild, untamed part of me. But here I was, stuck on the boat, unable to join these old men in their exploration. No one had bothered to tie me down this time, perhaps because I was now seen as nothing more than a fuck doll.

As the men adjusted their dive gear, they laughed and joked amongst themselves, making crude comments about my body and blonde hair. "Hey, did you hear the one about the blonde who tried to blow up her boyfriend's car?" one of them chuckled. "She burned her lips on the tailpipe!" The others roared with laughter, slapping each other on the back as they continued to share their lewd jokes. It was degrading, but somehow, I found myself enjoying the attention, even if it was demeaning.

Finally, the men were ready to dive. They slipped into the water one by one, leaving me alone on the boat with the captain, the dive-master, and the sound of the waves lapping against the hull. I peered longingly over the side, watching the bubbles rise to the surface as the group disappeared beneath the waves. The sun reflected off the water, casting shimmering patterns on the deck and teasing me with its beauty.

As I sat there, the sun beating down on my naked flesh, I couldn't help but fantasize about the return of the men, how they would use me once again, and what new depths of degradation we might explore together.

23

An Erotic Safety Stop

Naked and neglected, I lounged on the dive boat while the old men submerged themselves in the depths of the ocean. The captain and divemaster remained focused on their responsibilities, leaving me feeling like an abandoned toy.

I couldn't stand it anymore! Scuba diving had always been one of my passions, and I yearned to join them underwater, but there was no dive gear available for me.

I spotted a mask and snorkel lying on one of the benches. A devious grin spread across my face as I snatched them up, strapping the mask to my head and placing the snorkel between my eager lips. With a splash, I leaped from the platform at the back of the boat, embracing the cool water that enveloped my nude body.

As I swam at the surface, I mused to myself, "Maybe I'm a slave to the ocean, too!" Gliding through the water, I felt every subtle caress of the waves against my exposed skin, invigorating my senses and feeding my insatiable desire to be one with the sea. The first dive of the morning took the group on a deep dive, between 60 to 100 feet (18 to 30 m) below the surface. Though they were far beneath me, I could still see their location, thanks to the trail of bubbles rising to the surface.

With a sense of longing and determination, I swam toward the ascending bubbles, feeling the ocean's embrace as it caressed my nude form. The cool water glided over my young breasts, teasing my erect nipples, while the gentle current flirted with my thighs and the sensitive folds of my pussy. I felt more like an erotic animal than ever before, my primal desires amplified by the sensual touch of the sea.

As I reached the area where most of the bubbles were coming to the surface, I stopped and allowed myself to be enveloped by the sensations. Now, not only did the ocean's soothing touch tantalize my naked body, but the bubbles from the scuba divers' exhalation erotically massaged me as well. Bubbles tickled my perky breasts and sensuously brushed against my flat belly, making me shiver with delight. They playfully danced around my thighs, teasingly venturing closer and closer to my exposed, wet pussy.

I reveled in the intimacy of this moment, feeling connected to the men beneath me through their expelled breaths. With each bubble that grazed my skin, I was reminded of my purpose – to be one with the environment and fully embrace my role as a sex object for these old men. My mind buzzed with excitement, knowing that soon I would be reunited with the very source of these tantalizing bubbles.

The aquatic symphony of caresses continued, driving me into a state of heightened arousal. It was as if the ocean itself was conspiring to make me even more irresistible to the men I served. Their raw desires and hunger for my young body fueled my own lust, and I silently thanked the ocean for its part in this erotic dance. As I floated there, surrounded by a chorus of bubbles, I knew that no matter what happened next, I was exactly where I needed to be – a young, nude woman at the mercy of the sea and the older men who would soon return to claim her.

The scuba divers began to ascend slowly, heading towards a bar set up at 15 feet (5 m) from the surface for their safety stop. Because it was recreational scuba diving, the scuba divers did not need to do decompression stops. However, when diving below 60 feet, it is common practice to do a safety stop of at least 3 minutes at 15 feet (5 m).

As they gathered at the bar, their bubbles increased in intensity, massaging my body with greater assertiveness. From my vantage point, I could see the group huddled together, their minds surely in awe of the magical beauty of the underwater world they had just witnessed.

For me, the warm sun above and the cool water below formed an intoxicating contrast, heightening my senses and amplifying my arousal.

I hovered at the surface, watching as the men patiently completed their safety stop. My breath quickened with excitement, my heart pounding in my chest as I imagined the myriad ways they would use and abuse my body upon their return.

Eventually, some of the men looked up, and then, I could see their gazes locked on my exposed form, their eyes wide with hunger and admiration. The feeling of being an object of desire for these men filled me with a sense of purpose, reaffirming my belief in my role as a sex object for them to explore and indulge in their fantasies.

One of the divers signaled for me to swim down to their level. As an accomplished freediver and scuba diving instructor, I had no issue taking a deep breath, performing a graceful duck dive, and descending into the depths towards the group of scuba divers at 15 feet (5 m). The water hugged my naked body, amplifying my arousal and cementing my place in this underwater world as a sensual siren.

As I descended to join the group of 17 men at the 15-foot (5-meter) bar, their black wetsuits and scuba gear contrasted against my naked body, making my exposed skin stand out even more. My perky breasts and soft, round buttocks were illuminated by the sun's rays filtering through the water, drawing their hungry eyes to feast upon my vulnerable form.

As I reached the men, their stares intensified, and I reveled in the power and pleasure that my nudity offered. It was clear that I had captured their imaginations, and my presence within their midst only heightened their bestial cravings for sexual conquest.

One of the men, noticing my need for air, offered me his octopus, which I gratefully accepted. An octopus is the spare second stage of the regulator, allowing a buddy to breathe from the same scuba cylinder.

Unable to resist their primal urges, the old men began to play with my nude body. Fingers traced lines along my smooth skin, sending shivers of pleasure down my spine. Hands grasped at my tender breasts, pinching my nipples until they hardened in delight. Others ventured lower, caressing the delicate curves of my lower back and buttocks before daring to push into my wet, welcoming pussy.

I reveled in the sensations, my body arching and writhing under their touch. Each intimate stroke only served to further cement my role as a sex object for these men to use and enjoy. The cool water around us made every touch more pronounced, heightening my arousal and deepening my submission.

As their hands continued to explore my body, I couldn't help but feel intoxicated by the power they held over me. Their fingers pushed deeper into my most sensitive areas, eliciting gasps and moans from me as I tried to take in all the pleasure they offered.

Their bestial hunger for my flesh drove them on, each man seeking to leave his own mark upon my body.

A few of them attempted to slap my ass, but the resistance of the water made it difficult for them to do so with any force. The weak impacts produced little more than gentle ripples across my flesh, which only seemed to fuel their amusement further. A few of the men couldn't help but laugh at the situation, causing water to seep into their masks. They were forced to exhale deeply through their noses to clear the invading liquid, adding more bubbles to the surrounding water.

Meanwhile, I had nothing but my mask and the borrowed octopus to sustain me in the depths. My naked body was completely exposed and vulnerable, and I reveled in the attention and touch of the men around me.

With playful determination, a few of them took hold of my ankles and wrists, forcing me onto my back underwater. My supple breasts, composed mainly of fat tissue, floated upward in the most tantalizing way. The sight of my young boobs defying gravity and bobbing gently in the water captivated the men, who couldn't help but be fascinated by the alluring behavior of my buoyant mounds.

The contrast between their black wetsuits and scuba gear against the sheer vulnerability of my naked form only served to heighten the erotic atmosphere. Each man became more eager to explore and manipulate my body, driven by their bestial desires and insatiable lust for my youthful flesh. As they toyed with me in the depths, I embraced my role as their sexual plaything, allowing their touch to guide me deeper into submission.

Still held on my back by my ankles and wrists, I felt the men's grip tighten as they made their next move. One of them reached for my mask, pulling it off and leaving my eyes exposed to the salty sting of the ocean water. Another removed the octopus from my mouth, depriving me of my only source of air. Now completely nude and unable to breathe, I felt an exhilarating mix of vulnerability and arousal.

As my young, naked body floated in the depths, my inability to breathe only heightened the eroticism of the scene. I could feel the men staring at me, their gazes intense and hungry as they admired my perfect young form, reveling in the power they held over me.

Beneath the surface, the sight of my nude, helpless body seemed to awaken something primal within them, a bestial urge to dominate and possess the tantalizing creature before them. Their hands roamed my body, exploring every curve and crevice as they sought to claim me entirely for their own pleasure.

In those moments without air, my thoughts turned to my freediving training. The ability to hold my breath underwater for up to five minutes was a skill I had honed over time, and now it was proving invaluable. As seconds ticked by, I embraced the sensation of being at the mercy of these men, my lungs burning with the need for air but refusing to give in.

Finally, one of the men took pity on me and placed the octopus back into my mouth. I exhaled forcefully to clear the second stage before taking a deep, shuddering breath of compressed air. As I inhaled, relief flooded through me, along with a renewed sense of submission. I belonged to these men, their desires dictating every aspect of my existence, and that thought sent a shiver of pleasure running through my body.

Unfortunately, the safety stop came to an end, and they gave me back the freedom to move.

With a determined expression, I removed the octopus from my mouth and began my ascent to the surface. As a skilled scuba diving instructor, I knew the importance of exhaling all the way up to prevent lung overexpansion injury. The compressed air in my lungs expanded with every inch I rose, and I made sure to let it escape gradually, filling the surrounding water with a steady stream of bubbles.

They, too, began to ascend, but I lingered at the surface for a while, savoring the weightless embrace of the water. It was the first time I'd managed to go underwater during this dive trip, and I longed to extend the experience of being in the ocean as much as possible.

One by one, the 17 old men climbed back onto the dive boat, leaving me behind in the gentle waves. I watched them from afar, soaking in the caress of the sea. Eventually, when they were all on board, I swam back to the ladder at the rear of the boat, my nude form cutting through the water like a sleek, erotic fish.

As I gripped the ladder's cold metal rungs and pulled myself up, I could feel the eyes of the men on me, taking in the sight of droplets cascading down my naked body. My long blonde hair clung to my breasts, emphasizing their perky contours. My nipples hardened under their gaze, the cool sea breeze teasing them mercilessly.

Once back on board, I stood before the men, blatantly displaying my dripping, tantalizing body, feeling both vulnerable and powerful. Their admiration and raw desire fueled a fire within me, satisfying my need to be worshipped and adored.

"Damn, girl," one of the men remarked, his eyes glued to my soaked figure. "Just when I thought you couldn't get any sexier, you go and prove me wrong."

"Seeing you climb up that ladder made me wish I had a camera," another chimed in. "I'd have loved to capture the way the water streamed down your ass like an erotic waterfall."

"Even Venus herself would be jealous of how you emerged from the ocean, babe," a third man said, grinning lasciviously as he took in my watery form.

Their crude comments filled me with a perverse sense of pride. My body was their playground, and I reveled in the knowledge that every inch of my wet, nude form drove them wild with desire.

My role as an erotic creature was being fulfilled before their very eyes, and I couldn't help but relish the intoxicating sensation it brought.

"Careful, boys," I teased, my voice dripping with sensuality as I sashayed across the boat deck. "You wouldn't want to wear yourselves out too soon, now would you? There's still plenty of time left to enjoy this little fuck doll of yours."

Their laughter mingled with the sound of waves lapping against the boat, filling the air with a mixture of amusement and anticipation. As I continued to bask in their attention and admiration, I couldn't help but feel a deep sense of satisfaction, knowing that my body – young, nude, and dripping wet – was the source of their ravenous hunger for violent, bestial sex.

24

Nude: Sex Slave, Dive Gear Slave, Abused Waitress & Wild Outdoor Animal

The sun was setting, casting a warm glow over the small Caribbean island as I walked along the sandy beach toward the main building of the dive resort. As I looked around, I felt exhilarated by the fact that I had organized this dive trip with 14 old men who shared my passion for scuba diving and my belief that I was born to be a sex toy for old men.

As a recap, my goal for the week-long trip was especially to be fed a semen-only diet. Yet, I knew they would find it hard to resist my young, female body because, well... In my experience, men have strong reactions to my body – my long blonde hair, blue eyes, flat belly, perky breasts that bounced just enough to drive any man wild, and, of course, my soft waxed skin begging to be touched.

However, upon arriving at the dive resort, the group of old men decided to take things to another level. Instead of allowing me to join them in their underwater adventures, they punished me for being a blonde cock tease by making me their nude dive gear slave, banned for using dive gear for myself. Stripped of my clothes, I had no choice but to submit to their desires, setting up and tending to their dive gear before and after each dive completely naked.

As I carried out my duties under the watchful eyes of the old men, I could feel their raw primal hunger for my young, exposed body. The weight of their gazes on my bare flesh made me feel alive. In those moments, I found myself becoming even more determined to please them, to let them unleash their wild sexual instincts upon me.

With every piece of dive gear I meticulously set up, rinsed, and hung to dry, I reveled in the knowledge that I was fulfilling my purpose as a sex object for these old men. I embraced their dominance over me without hesitation. In fact, I loved it!

A ROUTINE SET in for the whole week, and I found myself eagerly embracing my role as a nude dive gear slave. Every morning, I attended to the group of 14 old men known as my Owners, setting up their dive gear before the dives and taking care of it after the morning boat dives. In the afternoons, I did the same for the group of 17 other scuba divers at the resort.

While the men were scuba diving, I swam naked at the surface with only a mask and snorkel, like an erotic sea creature. My body glided through the water, my long blonde hair floating behind me and my perky breasts bobbing gently with each stroke. I knew the sight of my naked form fueled the men's desires, and I reveled in it.

When it was time for the divers to do their safety stop at 15 feet (5 m) deep for 3 minutes at the end of their dive, I joined them underwater, holding onto the bar set for the safety stop. Despite being surrounded by the vast ocean, I still felt a sense of confinement – vulnerable, exposed, and wholly at the mercy of these men.

As we floated together, the old men played with my young, naked body. Their experienced hands explored every inch of my flesh, pinching my nipples, stroking my smooth, waxed pussy, and squeezing my ass. I could feel their bestial hunger for me, and it sent a thrill racing through my veins.

Every day, I received between 14 and 21 loads of semen from the 14 men owning my body during the morning dives. And in the afternoon, on the dive boat, I got between 17 and 25 loads of semen from the other 17 divers. Men fed me their semen on the way to the dive site, during the surface interval, and on the way back to the dock.

"Open wide, sweetheart," one man would say as he guided his cock to my eager lips. I'd take him into my mouth, savoring the taste and texture of his warm seed as it filled me. Another man might tease me, saying, "You're such a good little cum bucket," before offering me his semen delivery hose.

"Make sure you swallow every drop," another man would instruct, watching intently as I eagerly gulped down his thick load. Each time I did, I felt a sense of satisfaction and pride in knowing that I was fulfilling my role as a sex toy for these old men and that I was willingly submitting myself to their control.

Throughout the week, I spent my days in this erotic haze, my body a canvas for the old men's lust and desire, and my mind consumed by the knowledge that I was their property. My entire existence revolved around pleasing them, being their nude dive gear slave, and sustaining myself on a semen-only diet. And in those moments, with each passing day, I knew that I had never been more alive... or more fulfilled.

At lunchtime and during dinner, I found myself assuming the role of a nude sculpture, exposed for all to see. I would kneel on a table in a submissive position, my body glistening from the day's mix of sweat and seawater. As the men approached, I felt their eyes roaming over my naked form, taking in every inch of me as if they were assessing a piece of art. Their hands would occasionally reach out to touch me – a gentle caress here, a pinch there – reminding me that I was their object, their possession.

EVENINGS at the dive resort brought a new task for me. The old men decided that I would serve as their nude waitress, catering to their every need. This arrangement made sense to everyone; after all, I was not a guest but rather a non-human sex object, more like a nude robot in the flesh. And so, each night, I worked as a nude waitress, bringing drinks and snacks to the men while the barman insisted that all tips go to him.

As I moved gracefully between the tables, my long blonde hair swaying with each step, I felt the weight of the men's gazes on my bare skin. Their lustful eyes seemed to drink me in, reveling in the sight of my young female flesh on display.

I knew that I belonged to these men, and I wouldn't have it any other way. I always had that fantasy of being auctioned off to the highest bidder, with no safe word to safeguard what would happen to me. But that is a different story!

My days and nights blurred together in a haze of sexual servitude, both above and below the water's surface. Working as a nude dive gear slave, a nude erotic sea animal, and a nude piece of furniture decorating the dive resort, I embraced my role as a living embodiment of these old men's raw desires.

ONE EVENING, as I resumed my role as a nude waitress, the old men seemed more emboldened than ever. They were eager to push my boundaries and relish in their dominance over me.

"Hey, Delisha, bring us another round!" one of them barked, clearly testing the limits of his control over me.

"Coming right up," I replied sweetly, ignoring the demeaning tone. As I turned to head back to the bar, I felt a sharp slap on my ass, making it jiggle enticingly. The men erupted into laughter as I suppressed a smile, enjoying the sensation.

"Damn, this blonde's got quite the ass, huh?" another man

remarked, grinning lewdly at me. "I bet she'd love it if we made her bend over for a better view."

"Or maybe she'd like a finger inside her tight little pussy," chimed in yet another, pushing his index finger deep inside me without warning. I gasped but didn't object and resumed walking towards the bar, feeling the emptiness he had left behind.

"Even better, how about a finger in that tight little butthole of hers?" suggested a fourth man, following through with his proposal and inserting his thick digit into my anus. My body tensed momentarily before relaxing, accepting the intrusion.

"Maybe we oughta pinch those perky nipples too – teach her a lesson for being such a cock tease," said another man, reaching out and pinching my nipples harshly. I bit my lip, trying not to moan despite the pain mixed with pleasure.

"Next time you're slow with our drinks, we'll have to slap that pretty face of yours," threatened one of the men, shaking his fist playfully.

"Would you like that, Delisha? A nice, hard slap across your beautiful face?" another taunted, leaning in close and smirking.

"Whatever pleases you, gentlemen," I responded, my voice wavering with arousal. Their cruel words and actions only fueled my desire to serve them further.

The night wore on, and the men continued making degrading jokes about me and other young women, their laughter ringing in my ears as they reveled in their power over me.

"Hey guys, what's the difference between a blonde and a mosquito? A mosquito stops sucking after you slap it!" This joke caused raucous laughter among the men, their eyes filled with lust as they stared at me, probably remembering the numerous slaps they had inflicted on my young, female, nude body.

As each crude joke passed their lips, I felt an inexplicable thrill course through me. These old men were degrading me, treating me like a mere sex object for their amusement – and I loved every moment of it. Their desires and fantasies became my purpose, driving me to embrace this life of submission and servitude.

~

AS THE WEEK PROGRESSED, I found myself falling into a routine of sorts. Every night, I would sleep in the nude on the beach, my body exposed to the elements and the eyes of the old men who made up my Owners and the other guests at the resort.

There were offers from some of them for me to use their cabins' showers or even sleep indoors, but I couldn't help but feel that this was a once-in-a-lifetime opportunity. To spend an entire week outdoors, naked and vulnerable, was exhilarating and liberating. I knew I might never have this chance again, so I insisted on remaining outside like a wild animal.

Each morning, as I woke up, I would find traces of semen on my body, evidence that some of the men had masturbated over my sleeping form during the night. It was a gross yet erotic realization that even while I slept, my body was still an object of desire for these men. I wondered why they wouldn't simply fuck me instead, but then it occurred to me that perhaps there was a fetishistic thrill in just ejaculating over the naked body of a young, nude woman like me. And so, I let it happen, never saying a word about it, allowing them to satisfy their desires in any way they chose.

I would awaken each day feeling a mixture of disgust and arousal at the sight of the sticky substance clinging to my skin, knowing that it came from the very men I served and pleased throughout the day. I would take a moment to examine my body, running my fingers over the patches of dried cum, noting where they had chosen to leave their marks – on my breasts, stomach, thighs, and even sometimes on my face.

I found it oddly satisfying to discover these marks and feel the weight of their adoration for my young body. I couldn't resist running my fingers over the sticky patches, feeling the mixture of rough sand and smooth semen beneath my fingertips. I became addicted to this process, spreading the semen around my skin the best I could as if it were some sort of magical elixir that would keep me youthful and desirable forever.

This ritual became a crucial part of my mornings, solidifying my role as a sex object and reminding me of my purpose on this trip.

Once I had tended to my daily ritual, I made my way to the ocean's edge, allowing the cool water to lap at my feet. With each step, I submerged myself deeper into the crystal-clear water, feeling the gentle waves wash away the remains of the previous night's debauchery. The sensation of the water moving against my naked flesh, teasing and caressing every inch of me, was intoxicating. It was as if nature itself was embracing me, welcoming me into its fold as a wild, untamed creature.

In the end, each morning spent on the beach, spreading semen across my body and washing it away in the ocean, only served to strengthen my resolve and dedication to being a wild, untamed creature for these men to worship. And I loved every moment of it.

25

An Erotic Night Dive

On Wednesday, at dinner time, the air was warm and humid, as it had been all week. The resort manager stood up, a smile on his face. "Alright, everyone, who wants to do a night dive?" he asked. Eleven men raised their hands, some from my owners' group and others from the additional seventeen divers. Noticing the hesitation in the eyes of those who didn't volunteer, I couldn't understand why some were so scared or apprehensive about night diving. To me, it was always the best experience; there were creatures you could only see under the cloak of darkness.

My body tingled with anticipation, and my nipples hardened from both the excitement and the slight breeze that brushed against my naked skin.

As I had done every day this week, I prepared the dive gear for the eleven men going on the night dive. My nude body glistened with sweat from the tropical heat, garnering attention and lustful glares from the surrounding men. They taunted me with demeaning comments about blondes, pussy, and young women, but I reveled in their crude humor and sexual remarks.

"Hey Delisha, do you think your pussy can glow in the dark like those fish we're hoping to see tonight?" one of the divers joked, causing raucous laughter to erupt around the table.

"Maybe," I replied playfully, smirking. "You'll have to join the night dive to find out." Secretly, I enjoyed being the center of their raw desires, knowing that they worshipped my body like a sacred temple.

"Delisha's tight little blonde girl's ass could probably guide us through the darkest depths," another man chimed in, licking his lips as he eyed my exposed flesh.

"Damn right," I thought, biting my lip and feeling a surge of arousal run through my body. I knew I was an object of desire for these men, and it thrilled me to no end.

As the group continued to make crude jokes and remarks, I focused on preparing the dive gear, ready to embark on another thrilling adventure.

THE BOAT'S engine roared to life as we set off toward the dive site, the salty sea spray kissing my naked skin. My owners and the other divers had already begun their crude banter, poking fun at me and making lewd remarks about my body.

"Hey Delisha, do you think your pretty little asshole can take all eleven of us tonight?" one man asked with a wicked grin.

"Only one way to find out," I replied coyly, trying to mask my excitement. The thought of being used by these men sent an electric thrill down my spine.

As the boat sliced through the waves, the men took turns fucking my ass and pussy, each one leaving their mark upon my eager body. Their hard cocks penetrated me relentlessly, fueling my insatiable hunger for their raw desires. They made sure to ejaculate in my mouth, feeding me my much-needed semen-only diet.

"Damn, this dumb blonde is truly a cum bucket," a diver laughed, pushing himself deeper inside me. I simply moaned in response, savoring the throbbing sensation of his old cock filling me up.

UPON REACHING THE DIVE SITE, the men donned their scuba gear while I slipped on my snorkeling mask, snorkel, and fins. I could hardly contain my anticipation as they disappeared beneath the water's surface, leaving me alone to swim above them like a sensual siren.

I followed their exhaled bubbles, feeling the gentle caress of each one against my naked body. It was an almost otherworldly experience, like being embraced by the ocean itself. The underwater lights carried by the divers helped me keep track of their movements, guiding me as I swam along with them.

Moments of underwater exploration were always magical for me, but it was the way these men treated me that truly made this trip exceptional. They worshipped my body, used me in ways I craved, and pushed me to explore my darkest desires.

The shallow depth of the night dive made it easy for me to duck dive and descend toward the men. When I reached them, their focus immediately shifted from the reef to my naked body. They moved their underwater lights away from the coral formations, illuminating every inch of me as if I were an exotic ocean creature they had never encountered before. The beams of light danced across my skin, casting mesmerizing shadows and highlights that accentuated my curves and contours.

I reveled in the attention, feeling like a goddess of the sea, adored and worshipped by these old men who couldn't resist the allure of my nude form. As I swam among them, they occasionally offered me air through their octopus, allowing me to stay submerged for longer periods. Other times, I would swim back to the surface to catch a breath before diving down again, eager to rejoin my admirers.

Each time I ascended or descended, the men's eyes followed my movements with rapt attention, taking in the erotic sight of my naked body gliding effortlessly through the water. My long blonde hair flowed behind me like a silken banner while my firm, perky breasts gently bobbed with each undulation of my body.

My every movement seemed to captivate them, from the way my toned thighs gracefully propelled me through the water to the sensual arch of my back as I reached for the surface. I could feel the heat of their desire rising around me, fueling my own lust and need for more.

This underwater world had been my playground for years, but on that day, it was also a place where I could fully embrace my role as a sex object for these men to admire and worship. And as our night dive continued beneath the moonlit sky, I knew that I would never forget the intoxicating blend of beauty, lust, and power that had unfolded beneath the waves.

Their hands reached out to caress my body, exploring every inch with a mixture of curiosity and hunger. They seemed drawn to the sway of my buttocks as I moved through the water, their fingers tracing its roundness before slipping between my legs to feel the soft flesh there. My breasts also proved irresistible to them, their palms gently cupping each mound as they brushed their thumbs over my hardening nipples.

The sensation of their touch was almost too much to bear, sending waves of pleasure coursing through me. I loved how their rough, calloused hands contrasted with the smoothness of my skin, heightening the sensations even more. As I continued to swim alongside them, I reveled in the feeling of their fingers gliding along my thighs, up to my hips, and across my stomach. My hair floated around me like a golden halo, adding to the otherworldly atmosphere that enveloped us all.

Whenever I returned to the surface for air, I noticed a slight stinging sensation on my skin. Glancing down, I saw tiny jellyfish caught in the glow of the divers' lights. Undeterred by the discomfort, I continued to follow the men, entranced by the beauty beneath the waves and the erotic energy that pulsed between us.

Back on the boat, I examined the red spots that marked where the jellyfish had touched me. It barely hurt, but I knew I needed to rinse off with fresh water. "I'll just wash off with the hose by the pool," I told the group casually, trying to downplay the incident.

"Hey, Delisha, I'll bring you some vinegar too. That should help with the sting," the captain offered, showing a rare moment of concern amidst our wild escapades.

"Thanks," I replied with a genuine smile, appreciating his thoughtfulness even as I prepared myself for another round of debauchery with these insatiable men.

THE MOON CAST a silvery glow on the water as we made our way back to the dock. Despite the jellyfish stings, the men showed no signs of slowing down in their pursuit of pleasure. It seemed as though the darkness had unleashed their inner beasts, transforming the wolves into insatiable werewolves.

"Alright, Delisha," one man growled, "time for some spit-roasting."

"Bring it on," I taunted, eager to continue pushing my boundaries and satisfying their raw desires.

I positioned myself on all fours, and the men circled around me like predators. One positioned himself behind me, gripping my hips tightly before plunging his cock deep into my ass. Another knelt in front of me, guiding his throbbing erection past my lips and into my mouth.

As they fucked me relentlessly, I reveled in the feeling of being used and objectified by these older men. Their hands roamed over my body, leaving trails of sweat and lust in their wake. The sounds of our moans, groans, and grunts filled the night air.

"Fuck, your tight little ass is incredible!" the man behind me exclaimed, pounding me with ferocity. "You're such a filthy slut, taking all these cocks like a pro!"

"Show her how it's done, boys," another cheered from the sidelines, waiting for his turn to indulge in the erotic feast that was my body.

One by one, the men took their turns using me as their personal fuck doll, each eager to assert their dominance and revel in the debauchery. As they ejaculated, they always aimed for my mouth, coating my tongue with their hot, salty seed. I swallowed it down eagerly, savoring the taste and texture of each unique offering.

"Your mouth is like a fucking cum bucket," one man chuckled as he withdrew from my lips, his cock still twitching from the force of his orgasm.

"Thanks," I replied with a wicked grin, "I do my best."

"Look at this tight young ass," one of them grunted, grabbing my buttocks and squeezing them firmly. "Just begging for a good pounding."

"Her tits are so perfect, it's a sin," another chimed in, his calloused fingers pinching and twisting my nipples as he chuckled at my moans of pain and pleasure.

Another one smirked as he grabbed a handful of my blonde hair and pulled my head back, forcing me to look up at him with wide, pleading eyes.

"Make sure you don't choke on it, little slut," he taunted before thrusting his thick member past my lips and into my eager mouth. I gagged slightly but quickly adjusted, taking him deeper and deeper as he slammed himself into my throat.

"Can't get enough of that old cock, can you?" another man asked, positioning himself behind me and ramming into my wet pussy without warning. I gasped and moaned around the cock in my mouth, my body shaking with each powerful thrust.

"Is that all you got?" I managed to taunt them between thrusts, my words muffled by the cock still filling my mouth. "Are you real men or just old geezers?"

"Watch your mouth, girl," one of them growled, slapping my ass hard, leaving a stinging red mark in its wake. "Or we'll make you regret it."

As I was being fucked hard, memories of my previous experiences surfaced, making me appreciate the warm tropical climate even more. I mused about how the sultry heat allowed men to fuck my naked body at night without me getting cold, unlike my previous escapades in snowstorms. The thought of palm trees only strengthened my resolve to endure this relentless onslaught.

"Keep fucking her, boys," one of the men encouraged, his eyes glued to the erotic sight before him. "Make her remember this night forever."

"Trust me," I panted, feeling another orgasm building within me but determined not to let it overtake me, "I'll never forget."

Throughout the ride, the men continued to take turns spit-roasting me, never showing any sign of slowing down. Their crude humor, demeaning comments, and voracious appetites only fueled my desire for more. As we finally neared the dock, I couldn't help but feel a twisted sense of satisfaction at having endured and even enjoyed this carnal marathon.

"Damn, Delisha," one man said, admiring my now thoroughly used body, "you're one hell of a fuck toy."

"Thank you," I purred, catching my breath and preparing for whatever new adventures awaited me on the shore.

26

Underwater Sex

The warm Friday afternoon at the dive resort found me standing near the pool, my naked body on display for all to see. The old men admired me like a living sculpture, their eyes wandering over every curve and crevice as they reminisced about the debaucherous week we had shared together.

"Damn, Delisha," one man chuckled, "we sure did fuck you senseless this week, didn't we?" His buddies laughed along, their predatory gazes lingering on my exposed flesh.

"True," another chimed in, "but we haven't fucked our little whore underwater yet. What do you say, boys?"

As I watched the men around the pool discuss their new plans, it became clear that they were determined to take our sexual escapades to a higher level – or depth! The 11 most adventurous among them decided that they would finally fulfill their desire to fuck me underwater – the same 11 who had gone on a night dive on Wednesday.

"Alright, Delisha," one of the old men said, his voice thick with anticipation, "we'll see you down at the beach. You better be ready for us."

I simply nodded, my heart pounding with excitement, and began my nude walk towards the beach. My breasts swayed gently with each step, drawing the gazes of not just my Owners but also the other old men at the resort. Their crude remarks and lascivious laughter filled the air, but it only served to fuel my own desires.

I waited for them at the beach. Eventually, the 11 men arrived, scuba gear on their backs and fins in their hands. This time, though, instead of their usual wetsuits, they wore only bathing suits – an indication that they planned to use their cocks underwater. As they approached me, one of them asked, "So, Delisha, what's the best way to have sex underwater? We want to make sure we do this right."

For the first time since they started discussing underwater sex, they actually asked me something about our escapades together. "Well," I began, trying to keep my voice steady despite my arousal, "the most important thing is to find a spot where we can kneel on the sandy bottom without harming marine life. There's a place nearby where we can do that."

As we ventured further along the beach, the men continued their usual raucous teasing and crude jokes. They spoke of their eagerness to ravage my body beneath the waves, treating me as nothing more than a sex doll for their amusement.

"Remember, boys," another man chimed in, "this little whore loves to worship our old cocks, so make sure she gets a good taste of each one underwater."

With that, we arrived at the designated spot along the shore. The sun beat down on my naked body as I stood before them, like a lamb awaiting to be slaughtered.

The scene was a tableau of raw, primal eroticism. Around a nude, young female body, there was a group of old men dressed in scuba gear, their bodies imposing and virile despite their age. I could feel the heat radiating from their lustful gazes, each one fixated on my perky breasts, smooth stomach, and waxed pussy. The anticipation of what was to come made my heart race.

"Alright, boys," I called out, breaking the silence that had settled over us. "This beach is perfect for what you have in mind. We can kneel on the sandy bottom without damaging any marine life." I pointed to the floating line that marked the boundary of the swimming area. "There's about 15 feet of water at the line furthest from shore. Trust me, I know – I've slept naked on this beach all week and swam in the ocean every morning."

The men exchanged knowing glances. One of them piped up, his voice rough and gravelly, "Well, aren't you just the perfect little sea nymph?"

Another chimed in, "We're gonna make sure you get a good taste of our saltwater gods, sweetheart."

As they continued making crude comments and jokes about the upcoming underwater adventure, I felt a thrill running through my veins. This was an entirely new experience, a chance for me to fulfill my role as their willing sex object while also indulging my passion for the ocean. And though I knew their intentions were far from noble, I relished the opportunity to be used and worshipped in such a unique, otherworldly setting.

"Hey, can one of you bring an extra weight belt for me?" I asked the group of old men as they prepared to enter the water. "And don't forget to share your air with me every once in a while, okay?"

"Of course, baby girl," one of them replied with a grin. "Can't have our sexy little mermaid suffocating down there."

"Alright, let's do this!" I shouted, feeling my excitement grow as we all swam out to the floating line that marked the boundary of the swimming area.

As we reached the spot, the men began to descend, forming a circle on the sandy bottom. The anticipation was palpable – it felt like we were about to participate in some ancient, forbidden ritual. I took a deep breath and performed a graceful dock dive, my naked ass and legs momentarily soaring through the air before I plunged into the water.

I swam down to join the circle of eager old men, my bare body on full display for their lecherous gazes. I signaled to the diver who had brought the spare weight belt, and he handed it to me. I secured it on my legs while I knelt down in the center of the circle.

One of the men offered me his octopus – the spare second stage of his regulator – and I gratefully accepted it, breathing deeply from the shared air source. There I was, completely nude and vulnerable, surrounded by a group of old men ready to use and worship me in this surreal underwater setting.

Submerged in the clear ocean water, I found myself at ease despite the situation. I hadn't bothered to bring a mask, believing it would only interfere with the blowjobs I intended to give these old men. I'd never understood why some people had difficulty opening their eyes underwater – it came naturally to me, both in the sea and in swimming pools.

As we settled into our positions, I noticed that nobody was making a move. Perhaps they were uncertain about how to initiate this underwater orgy, or maybe they were simply savoring the sight of my naked body on display for them. Regardless, I decided to take charge, giving them a crude sign with my hands: I formed a circle with my thumb and index finger on one hand while thrusting the index finger of my other hand in and out of the loop.

I could hear muffled laughter through the second stages of their regulators, the sound distorted by the water. It seemed my vulgar gesture had broken the ice, and the anticipation among the group grew more intense.

I went on all fours while a diver finally approached me from behind, taking advantage of my vulnerable position. As he began to thrust into my exposed pussy, I noticed an odd sensation – the water resistance slowed his movements, making the usual rhythm of our copulation feel strange and unfamiliar.

Even so, there was something undeniably erotic about the situation. Here I was, a nude young woman at the mercy of these old men, surrounded by a circle of their eager stares as they watched the action unfold. The scene was charged with raw sexual energy.

The feeling of being used and objectified only added to the

intensity of the moment, feeding my own perverse desire to be completely submissive to their lustful whims. In that underwater world, my sole purpose was to satisfy these men's carnal needs, and I reveled in playing the role of their willing underwater fuck doll.

While one man continued to pump into me, I could sense the others watching. I knew that my naked body, caressed by water and illuminated by the filtered sunlight streaming down from above, must have been an intoxicating sight for these men who had spent so much time exploring the depths of their bestial desires throughout the week.

Each thrust pushed me further into the warm sand beneath me, and I couldn't help but imagine how it would feel to be completely buried in its embrace while being fucked so passionately. The thought only served to heighten the eroticism of the situation, and I found myself craving more – to be devoured by these men, to become the embodiment of their most primal urges.

As I surrendered myself to the relentless pounding from behind, my body quivered with each movement, sending ripples through the water around us. In that moment, I was both a part of the ocean's vast expanse and entirely separate from it, a living testament to the power of human lust and desire.

As the man behind me continued to pound my pussy, I felt an insatiable urge to take things even further and do something I had done many times before but only in a pool – sucking a cock underwater. The first time was at my hometown's local dive shop, and I took a liking to it. But this would be my first time doing it in the ocean, where I felt most alive and connected with my deepest desires. And I gotta say, I much prefer the taste of salt than that of chlorine!

With a determined glint in my eye, I signaled for the man providing me air from the octopus to come closer. He understood what I wanted and moved towards me, anticipation radiating from his body. As he approached, I reached for his waistband and pulled down his bathing suit, exposing his semi-erect cock to the caressing seawater.

Taking a deep breath from the octopus, I removed it from my mouth and eagerly took his hard rod between my lips. Letting out a steady exhale, I pushed the seawater out of my mouth while sealing my lips around his hard rod. The sensation was unlike anything I had ever experienced before – the saltiness of the water still lingering in my mouth only served to heighten the eroticism of the act.

As I began to work my tongue around his stiff cock, my mind wandered to the crude jokes they had made throughout the week, objectifying me and treating me as nothing more than a sexual plaything for their amusement. In this moment, I felt like a living embodiment of those jokes, a testament to the power of their bestial desire for my young woman's body.

The taste and texture of his shaft in my mouth brought forth memories of all the other men who had taken me this week, each one leaving their mark on me in their own unique way. I found myself reminiscing about the way they worshiped my naked form, treating their old cocks as gods to be revered by my youthful, submissive body.

My head bobbed up and down in rhythm with the man's slow thrusts, the water resistance forcing us to take our time with each movement. I focused on keeping my lips sealed around his erection, ensuring no seawater seeped in while I pleasured him. My senses were heightened, my entire world reduced to the feeling of his cock in my mouth and the taste of his pre-cum as it mixed with the remnants of seawater that still lingered on my tongue.

The scene unfolding before me was one of pure eroticism – my nude body surrounded by a circle of old men, each one watching intently as I knelt on the ocean floor, performing an underwater blowjob that would forever be etched into my memory.

The sensation of underwater sex was like nothing I had ever experienced before. As the man who had been fucking my pussy withdrew, I could only guess that he had reached his climax and released his seed inside me. The water around us made it difficult to discern the exact moment, but that didn't matter – what mattered was the raw pleasure we were all indulging in.

Another man took his place behind me, eager to continue this erotic underwater ritual while I persisted in sucking the cock in front of me, my tongue dancing around the shaft as I savored the taste of him – an extra salty version of it. Every now and then, I would need to pause for a breath, removing the cock from my mouth to take the octopus and purge the water from it. I'd inhale deeply, then return my attention to the erection waiting patiently for me.

This process was time-consuming, yet somehow, it only added to the thrill of our aquatic rendezvous. Each breath felt like a stolen moment, a brief respite before plunging back into the depths of debauchery that surrounded me. The men watched intently, their eyes filled with lustful hunger as they admired my naked form, worshipping my body like the divine offering it was.

My body quivered under their touch, a mix of excitement and the ever-present chill of the ocean water caressing my skin. My nipples stood erect, goosebumps covering my body as I surrendered myself to the experience. I reveled in the knowledge that I was their toy, their object of lust and desire, existing solely for their pleasure.

This underwater orgy was like nothing I'd ever experienced before, and it got worse (I mean, better). With a firm grip on my neck, a man pushed my face into the sand below while thrusting his cock in my butthole. I closed my eyes tightly, trying to keep the sand out. The octopus providing me with air slipped from my mouth as my face was forced down, leaving me breathless.

I couldn't breathe or see anything, but the erotic sensation of being abused underwater by this man sent shivers throughout my body. This bestial display of dominance was exactly what I craved – to be used and treated like an object for their pleasure. My naked body, vulnerable and exposed, was at the whim of these men and their raw desires.

The man continued pounding into my butthole with no regard

for my comfort or safety. It was as if he wanted to punish me for being so tempting, so irresistible to him and the others. And in that moment, I felt more alive than ever despite the lack of oxygen. As my mind teetered on the edge of consciousness, I reveled in the carnal nature of the scene unfolding around me. This was where I belonged, a young nude woman being taken and claimed by these men.

In the midst of the underwater chaos, I knew the other men were watching, waiting for their turn to use me as they pleased.

My body, the centerpiece of this primal dance, was both my prison and my sanctuary. The feeling of being completely at their mercy, unable to escape or resist, was intoxicating.

Somewhere deep within me, a small voice whispered that it was wrong – that I should fight back, demand my freedom, and find air to breathe. But the louder, more insistent part of me drowned out those thoughts, reveling in the eroticism of the moment. This was what I had chosen, and I wouldn't trade it for anything.

The man behind me, ruthlessly pounding my ass, held a divine power over me. He controlled my very existence as my body writhed and thrashed helplessly in the sand. My naked form was a sacrificial flesh offering to these old men, their lustful desires consuming me like a ravenous beast.

As the urge to breathe became unbearable, I struggled to remain conscious. My mind desperately clung to the sensations around me: the grit of the sand against my face, the salty water engulfing my submerged body, and the relentless thrusts filling my ass. Each detail served as a reminder of the dark, primal desire of these cock-carrying animals.

Suddenly, I felt a touch on my cheek, followed by a firm grip on my hair. The man yanked my head up, and I felt something familiar pressed against my lips – the mouthpiece of an octopus. Desperate for air, I took it between my lips, purging it and tasting the sweet relief of air as I breathed in deeply.

Despite the respite, the other man didn't pause for a second. He continued to pound my ass mercilessly, each thrust sending jolts of pleasure mixed with pain through my body. As I took in this much-needed breath, my thoughts raced.

I realized how truly vulnerable I was, trusting these men with my life as well as my body.

My heart pounded violently in my chest, a mix of fear and arousal coursing through my veins. It was a cruel paradox, knowing that my survival hinged on the whims of men who only saw me as a piece of meat to be devoured. This realization only heightened the experience, adding an intoxicating edge to the eroticism of the situation.

Still floating underwater, my body aching from the relentless pounding I'd received in my ass, I felt another pair of hands on me. The man behind me slipped out, leaving my butthole throbbing and empty. Suddenly, I was flipped onto my back by another man, my long blonde hair billowing around me like a mermaid's tail.

As I adjusted to the new position, I realized that being underwater made it so much easier for these men to maneuver me however they pleased. Their strong hands gripped my body, asserting their dominance over me, and I reveled in it.

This man positioned himself between my legs, pushing them apart as he knelt down. He lined up his cock with my aching pussy and thrust inside, filling me completely. My body floated horizontally in the water, my head tilted slightly upward. I marveled at how effortlessly these older men could manipulate me in this environment, even those who didn't possess particularly impressive physiques.

The scene was erotic in its raw, bestial nature: my naked young body floated horizontally in front of this man while he fucked my pussy mercilessly. My breasts, primarily composed of fat, tried to float toward the surface, wobbling comically with each powerful thrust. It seemed as though they were dancing in the water, a playful contrast to the carnal act taking place between my legs.

As my body continued to bounce and sway with each thrust, I couldn't help but feel a strange sense of pride in how easily I had given myself over to these men. And despite the intense sensations coursing through my body, I remained steadfast in my commitment not to orgasm, determined to deny myself that ultimate release. The thought of these old men using my body as they saw fit, without any regard for my own pleasure or satisfaction, only served to heighten the eroticism of the situation. I had truly become a sacrificial lamb, my body offered up on the altar of their lust and desire.

Surrounded by a group of old men in scuba gear, I continued to float horizontally underwater while the men took turns between my legs. The sensation of being completely naked and vulnerable as they stared at my exposed body only added to the eroticism of the situation.

The men reached out with their wrinkled hands to grope and play with my naked boobs. Their rough, greedy fingers pinched and squeezed my nipples, sending jolts of arousal through my body. Their eyes feasted on the sight of my helpless form, taking in every inch of my young flesh.

This bestial display of lust had a strangely alluring quality; these old men took turns to fuck me while they toyed with my boobs, treating me like an underwater fuck doll. It was evident that they found great delight in watching my breasts trying to float toward the surface, bouncing and quivering with each powerful thrust.

As one man finished, another eagerly took his place, continuing the relentless pounding into my willing pussy. My body remained floating horizontally, making it easy for them to switch positions without having to exert any effort.

In the midst of this underwater orgy, I concentrated on the sensations coursing through me – the coolness of the ocean contrasting with the heat of the men's bodies and the mixture of pain and pleasure from being used so roughly. Despite the intense feelings, I regularly reminded myself not to climax, determined to remain a true sex object for their enjoyment.

The eroticism of the situation intensified when, every so often, one of the men would yank the octopus from my mouth, leaving me gasping for air. My life was truly in their hands, and each time they pulled the mouthpiece away, I felt a thrill of fear mixed with excitement. They teased me mercilessly, keeping the octopus just out of reach as I struggled to grab it.

As I writhed beneath them, my body aching from the non-stop pounding, I lost all sense of time. The underwater world around me seemed to fade into the background, my entire focus narrowing down to the relentless rhythm of their cocks thrusting into me and the cruel game they played with my air supply.

Eventually, a man fucking my pussy withdrew his cock, and no one took his place. For a moment, I thought the underwater orgy had come to an end. But instead of allowing me to swim to the surface, the men continued toying with my nude body, running their rough hands over my tender flesh and occasionally granting me a precious breath from the octopus. Each denied breath sent a jolt of panic through me, heightening my arousal even further.

With my lungs begging for air, I couldn't help but revel in the degradation and humiliation I was subjected to. This perverse underwater game brought me to the edge of ecstasy while simultaneously reminding me of my role as a sex object for these old men to use as they pleased.

As I floated there, completely at their mercy, pushed around like an underwater beach ball, I realized that this was precisely what I craved – the feeling of being utterly powerless. The knowledge that my very life depended on their whims only served to deepen my desire to submit to their every demand.

At last, the men seemed to tire of their cruel game, and I was permitted to swim to the surface. My body bore the marks of their abuse, but my spirit soared with dark and twisted satisfaction.

The moment I finally reached the surface, gulping in the warm, salty air, I felt a bizarre mix of relief and disappointment. My body was sore and exhausted from the underwater orgy, but at the same time, I couldn't deny that part of me craved more, yearning for the relentless abuse and degradation that only some men were willing to provide.

"Look at our little fishy, gasping for air," one man chuckled as they swam up beside me, their eyes glittering with cruel amusement. "Did you enjoy being choked without even having a cock in your mouth?"

I blushed at his words, knowing full well how much I had enjoyed the feeling of helplessness and vulnerability that came from being unable to breathe. These men held the power of life and death over me, and it thrilled me beyond measure.

Once we reached the shore, the men carelessly tossed their dive gear onto the sand, ordering me to carry it all back to the dive shop, rinse it to thoroughly remove sand and salt, and hang it to dry. As I bent down to pick up the first set of equipment, my naked body on full display, I felt a surge of excitement as I realized what lay ahead. Each trip to the dive shop meant another walk past the bar where the men would be relaxing, sipping their drinks, and undoubtedly waiting to catcall and whistle at their nude dive gear slave.

With each trip, the weight of the scuba gear seemed to grow heavier, but I reveled in the task, feeling the strain on my muscles and the lingering ache between my legs as a reminder of the debauched acts I had just endured. The crude comments and lascivious stares from the men only served to heighten my arousal, and I found myself smiling coyly in response, basking in their admiration and lust.

"Hey, baby girl!" one of the men called out as I walked by, struggling under the weight of yet another set of dive gear. "You're doing a great job, sweetheart. But I think you could use a little more weight. How about carrying my cock around in that tight little pussy of yours?"

His words sent a thrill through me, and I couldn't help but let out a soft moan as I imagined his thick cock buried deep inside me, filling me up completely as I continued to serve these men like the sex slave and dive gear slave they had turned me into.

"Maybe later," I replied with a teasing wink, knowing that there was still time for more play time on our last day of this unforgettable week of debauchery and submission. With each step I took, my body swayed provocatively, every curve on display for their enjoyment. And as I basked in their hungry gazes, I knew without a doubt that I belonged to them – a willing offering to the gods of old cocks, destined to be used and abused for their pleasure alone.

27

Beer Mugs, Semen Mugs & Pee Mugs

On the last Saturday, we spent most of the time at the bar because there was no diving scheduled in the last 24 hours before the flight back home. And on that day, men had decided that they wanted to see the blonde, nude chick drink semen out of a beer mug.

With the help of the barman, they collected semen. Even though it was a group of old men, they managed to produce quite a lot of ejaculation. I'm guessing that Viagra and the sight of my naked body helped!

Now that I am sitting here to write this part of my sex diary, I'm wondering how the barman maintained the semen while collecting it. I should have asked!

~

AS THE OLD men circled around me, their lustful eyes fixated on my naked body, I felt a sense of exhilaration. They had brought with them a large beer mug filled to the brim with their collective semen.

I am addicted to semen. I need it! Yet, the viscous liquid in that beer mug appeared disgusting and repulsive, with its uneven texture and off-white hue. A pungent scent wafted from the mug, sharply contrasting with the sweet aroma of tropical cocktails that lingered in the air.

"Alright, Delisha, time for you to chug this down," one of the men commanded, his voice dripping with authority. I could see the anticipation in their faces, the eagerness to see me, their sex slave, obey without hesitation. With a smirk, I took the heavy mug into my hands, feeling the warmth of the contents inside.

As I raised the brimming mug to my lips, I could feel the gazes of the old men burning into my skin. The thought of gulping down their thick, salty seed was exhilarating, and I felt aroused by the power they held over me. In my mind, I embraced my role as their sex pet and the belief that consuming their semen was simply part of my natural diet.

Taking a deep breath, I tilted the mug back and began to chug the viscous liquid. And I got quite a surprise! I love the taste of semen coming out of a man's cock. But what I drank out of that beer mug tasted just as disgusting as it looked, with an overpowering saltiness and an oddly bitter aftertaste. I felt my throat muscles working as I swallowed mouthful after mouthful, the substance sliding down my gullet like warm, slimy oysters.

At first, the room was silent, except for the wet sounds of my gulping and the occasional hushed snicker from the men. My chest heaved with effort as I struggled to consume the entire mug without stopping.

As I kept drinking, some old men looked disgusted by the sight before them, unable to hide their grimaces and turned away faces, while others stared with morbid fascination at the remnants of their own seed smeared across my lips. And yet, most old men's eyes gleamed as they watched the disgusting concoction disappear into my mouth, their dumb blonde sex slave eagerly obeying their every command.

"Never thought I'd see the day when someone would actually drink that shit," one muttered, shaking his head in disbelief as he wiped sweat from his brow.

"Me neither," agreed another, his voice laced with a mixture of awe and repugnance. "It's just... so wrong."

"Yet, strangely erotic," a third added, smirking as he glanced at me, his eyes taking in every inch of my exposed flesh as if trying to memorize the sight of me for later.

As I stood there, a sticky, debased mess and the object of their twisted desires, I couldn't help but feel a perverse sense of satisfaction. In that moment, I was exactly what they wanted – a beautiful, dumb blonde who would submit to their every depraved whim without question or complaint.

"Look at her," one of them whispered with a smirk, "taking it all down like the little cum-guzzling bimbo she is."

As I finally drained the last drops from the mug and set it down with a triumphant thud, I couldn't help but feel a perverse sense of pride. I had proven myself as their obedient pet, willing to indulge in even the most depraved acts for their satisfaction. With semen still coating my lips and tongue, I looked up at the grinning faces surrounding me, knowing that I had given them exactly what they craved – complete control over a young, beautiful woman – a dumb blonde – who would do anything to please them.

"Isn't she just perfect?" an old man said, his eyes devouring my naked form, lingering on my heaving breasts and the lewd mess still smeared across my face. "She's everything we could've wanted – and more."

"Good girl," chimed in another one, reaching out to stroke my cheek almost affectionately, though his tone was anything but gentle. "But you know what they say – you need something to wash it down."

"Right," agreed the first man, snapping his fingers as if struck by sudden inspiration. "A nice cold beer should do the trick."

"Or something even more fitting for our lovely little cum dumpster here," a male voice dripping with cruel amusement proposed. He glanced around the room as if seeking approval from his companions.

When he saw the wicked grins spreading across their faces, he gave a nod and unzipped his pants. As he took out his cock, two others followed suit without hesitation. The sight of these old, powerful cocks—each a god that I longed to worship—made my heart race even faster. They were more than ready to show me just how low they thought of me.

"Let's give our dumb blonde a little treat, eh?" one of them said, his voice dripping with crude mockery. "I bet she can't wait to down this."

Chuckling and exchanging lewd remarks, the men filled a new beer mug with their warm, yellow piss. Each stream added to the growing volume, creating a concoction that I knew I would soon be forced to drink. Their laughter grew louder, their taunts harsher, as they reveled in my degradation.

"Look at her," another man snickered. "It matches the color of her hair. She was born for it."

My mind spun with conflicting emotions as they continued to fill the mug. Part of me recoiled from the idea of drinking their urine, but another part of me—the part that craved submission and debasement—was eager to prove myself to them. To show them that I was indeed the sex slave they desired and that nothing would stop me from satisfying their twisted appetites.

As the last few drops fell into the now-brimming mug, they stepped back, admiring their handiwork. One of the men handed me the mug. The pungent aroma invaded my nostrils, causing me to shudder involuntarily.

"Here you go, sweetheart," he said with a wicked grin. "Drink up and show us just how much of a dumb blonde you really are."

I took a deep breath, steeling myself for what was to come. I lifted the mug to my lips, my hands shaking ever so slightly from both anticipation and trepidation.

"Bottoms up," I murmured, offering them a sultry smile as I tilted the mug back and began to chug.

The men watched with bated breath when I began to drink their vile concoction, determined to prove that I was everything they wanted me to be—and more.

As I continued to chug the foul concoction, I could see the expressions on some of the old men's faces twisting in disgust. The sight of me downing the beer mug filled with their urine seemed to both repulse and intrigue them. Their eyes were glued to my face, watching as a little bit of the yellow liquid trickled down my chin and splashed onto my bare chest, finding a way between my young tits. It was clear they found the content revolting, yet they couldn't tear their gazes away from the erotic spectacle.

Despite the sickening taste and humiliation of the situation, I felt a perverse thrill at being so utterly degraded by this group of men. As their sex slave, it was my duty to obey their every command – no matter how vile or demeaning. I knew that by drinking their pee, I was further proving myself to be the dumb blonde they wanted me to be. And in some twisted way, that thought only fueled my desire to please them even more.

With every swallow, I could sense their arousal growing, their lust for me intensifying as they reveled in my degradation. It was intoxicating – like a drug that made me crave more. I took perverse pride in my ability to satisfy their darker desires, pushing myself to endure the humiliation for their pleasure.

Finally, I drained the last drop from the mug, my throat burning from the acrid taste. As I lowered the empty mug, gasping for breath, I met their eyes – searching for any hint of approval or satisfaction in their lecherous gazes.

And there it was, that unmistakable glint of raw desire and lustful appreciation that confirmed what I already knew: I had succeeded in pleasing them. My obedience and willingness to degrade myself for their amusement had only served to fuel their erotic fantasies.

My body, my very existence, was reduced to a mere plaything for these older men. And in that moment, I realized just how much I reveled in my role as their dumb blonde sex slave – the object of their darkest, most primal desires.

28

Father's Day Spankings for a Naughty Girl

As I woke up on the beach, I felt the familiar sensation of dried semen on my naked body. My skin was coated in a thin layer of salty evidence from the men who had pleasured themselves over me while I slept. The sun was just rising, casting a warm glow on my bare skin.

I loved finding these cum tributes on my body every morning – it reminded me of the pictures I'd seen online where men would ejaculate over pictures of girls. But this was so much better; these men were using my actual body as their canvas!

Sitting up on the sand, I admired the erotic sight of my young, nude body covered with their offerings. Sand had stuck to the dried semen, giving me an appealingly dirty appearance that only enhanced my allure. My firm, perky breasts bore traces of their lust, and I couldn't help but feel a thrill at being used in such a primal way.

My naked buttocks pressed against the gritty sand, reminding me that I wasn't deserving of a comfortable bed or shower. No, I was meant to be a wild, untamed creature, existing solely for the pleasure of these older men who craved my youthful body.

I waded into the ocean, the cool water washing away the

remnants of semen and sand from my naked body. The waves lapped at my skin, a cleansing caress that rid me of the evidence of the debauchery. I submerged myself completely, rinsing my long, tangled blonde hair in the salty water. After a week of sleeping outdoors with no shower, it was a tangled mess, but I reveled in the wild, untamed feeling it gave me.

Emerging from the ocean, I headed back to the resort's outdoor breakfast area. My nude body glistening with water droplets, I walked confidently among the guests, knowing full well the impact my exposed form had on the older men around me. I felt their hungry eyes devouring every inch of my nakedness, and it sent a wicked thrill through me.

Upon reaching the buffet, I stood next to it like a piece of art since I was not allowed to eat anything other than the semen from old cocks. It was then that I remembered: it was Father's Day. A wicked smile spread across my face as I recalled the plan we'd devised for this special occasion.

"Harvey," I said, finding him among the crowd of men, "remember our plan for Father's Day? All the men who are old enough to be my father were supposed to give me a spanking if they thought I'd been a bad girl."

His eyes lit up with dark amusement, and he glanced around at the others before responding. "Oh, I think we can all agree that you've been very bad, Delisha."

My heart raced with anticipation, eager to submit to these older men and let them unleash their most primal desires upon my willing body. For today, I would be their object of lust and punishment, a living canvas for them to leave their marks on. And I couldn't wait to see just how far they would go.

"Alright, gentlemen," Harvey announced as he whistled loudly to gather their attention. "Today's a special day, and our little Delisha here has reminded me that she's been quite the bad girl on this trip." He looked around at the group of 14 men who owned me, as well as the 17 other divers who were also old men. Nods and murmurs of agreement filled the air.

"Since it's Father's Day, I think it's only fitting that any man old enough to be her father should give her a spanking – teach her some manners before we head back home." A chorus of approving grunts and laughter followed his words, and I couldn't help but feel both excited and nervous at the prospect of being at the mercy of these older, experienced men.

"Let's start with a demonstration, shall we?" Harvey said, pulling up a chair and forcing my nude body onto his knees. My heart pounded in anticipation as my hair dangled down, whipping the floor, and my breasts swayed beneath me. I felt their eyes glued to my vulnerable form, each one clearly eager to take part in my punishment.

"Delisha, you've been a very bad girl, teasing us all week with that tight little body of yours," Harvey scolded, his voice firm and commanding. "It's time you learned your place."

With that, he brought his hand down hard on my bare ass, causing me to gasp and wince in pain. I could almost feel the men growing more aroused by the spectacle. The stinging sensation sent a mix of pain and pleasure coursing through me, and I knew that this was just the beginning of a long, torturous ordeal.

"Come on, harder!" one of the men shouted from the crowd. "Make sure she learns her lesson, for real!"

Harvey obliged, his hand landing on my ass with even more force. Tears already threatened to well up in my eyes as the pain intensified, but I refused to cry out or plead for mercy. I wanted this. I needed this. And I knew that every man watching me was just as hungry for the sight of my punished flesh as I was for their rough touch.

"Remember, gentlemen," Harvey said through gritted teeth as he continued to spank me mercilessly, "today is the day we show her who's in charge. Don't hold back."

As I lay across his knees, my body trembling from the relentless punishment, I couldn't help but revel in the knowledge that I was giving these men exactly what they craved – the chance to dominate and control a young, beautiful woman like myself. And I couldn't wait to see just how far they would push me in their quest to satisfy their darkest desires.

With the men cheering and encouraging Harvey, he kept hitting my buttocks hard while explaining to the crowd that he expected them to be just as rough so that I, the young blonde whore and bad girl, learned a lesson. The pain intensified with each strike, but it only fed my craving for humiliation and punishment.

"Alright, Harvey, let someone else have a go!" Fred shouted, stepping forward with a devilish grin on his face. "I've got a better idea to make sure she really feels this."

Fred suggested a different way to give me a series of spankings: he wanted me to bend over with my ass up in the air, and then he wanted to tie my wrists to my ankles. Harvey helped Fred do it, and as they secured the knots, I could feel my vulnerability increasing. My exposed position left nothing to the imagination, and I knew that all the men were enjoying the sight of my naked body displayed before them like a punching bag.

It seemed the scene of a young nude female tied like that was incredibly erotic for the old men. They gazed hungrily at my round ass, now red from the spanking, and the way my breasts dangled down, swaying with every slight movement. My long, messy blonde hair fell forward, brushing against the floor beneath me and framing my flushed face.

"Look at her," one man said, licking his lips. "She's like a present, all wrapped up and waiting for us to unwrap her." The others laughed and nodded in agreement, their eyes never leaving my body.

"Damn right," another chimed in. "I'd love to take her home like this."

The crude jokes and lewd remarks only served to heighten my arousal, even as I braced myself for the brutal spankings that were to come.

"Alright, boys," Fred said, cracking his knuckles. "Let's make sure she never forgets this Father's Day."

Fred's hands were eager to deliver the next round of punishment. I could see the excitement in his eyes as he positioned himself behind me. The old men surrounding us watched intently, their lustful gazes glued to my nude body tied up and presented for their entertainment.

"Keep that ass up, Delisha," Fred commanded, his voice rough and authoritative. I obeyed, pushing my hips back and arching my spine to present my reddened ass even more prominently. The men let out approving grunts and murmurs, clearly aroused by my submissive posture.

"Look at her," one man said, chuckling. "She's just begging for it."

With a swift motion, Fred brought his hand down on my already sore buttocks. The impact was so forceful that it pushed me forward, causing me to stumble slightly. My wrists strained against the ties binding them to my ankles, making it difficult to maintain my balance. The men found my struggle amusing, laughing and making crude remarks about how much I must be enjoying the pain.

"Doesn't she look like a wild animal, all tied up like that?" another man commented. "It's like we're breaking her in, showing her we own her."

"Damn right," agreed another. "She needs to learn her place – on her knees, worshipping our cocks."

As Fred continued to spank me with increasing force, the scene only grew more erotic for the old men. They reveled in my vulnerability, delighting in the way my breasts swung and jiggled with each punishing blow. My body glistened with sweat, the salty droplets mingling with the remnants of semen from earlier, leaving trails down my skin.

The third man couldn't wait any longer and retrieved a wooden spatula from the buffet table. He grinned wickedly as he brandished the makeshift instrument of discipline. "Time to really teach this little tease a lesson," he said, his eyes gleaming with anticipation.

He took his place behind me and swung the spatula down onto my dark red ass cheeks. The sting was more intense than before, making me gasp and whimper in pain. But even through the agony, I couldn't deny the twisted satisfaction I felt as their object of desire, their perverse plaything.

"Look at that ass," someone exclaimed. "Can't wait to see how red it gets after we're done with her."

"Best Father's Day gift ever," another chimed in, laughing heartily.

The men took turns spanking my naked ass with the wooden spatula, each one eager to make their mark on my reddening flesh. My head hung low, and I felt dizzy from the position and the relentless barrage of pain. Every so often, my legs would buckle, and I'd collapse onto my side on the ground.

"Get her back up," one man ordered, his voice gruff and commanding.

A couple of the men grabbed my hips and hauled me back into the degrading position, my wrists still tied to my ankles. Despite the discomfort and humiliation, I couldn't deny the dark thrill that coursed through me at being so completely objectified and controlled by these old men.

"Look at you, such a bad girl," one man taunted as he whacked the spatula across my ass, making me yelp in pain. "You deserve every bit of this punishment."

"Maybe after we're done, you'll learn to be a better whore for us old men," another chimed in, his voice dripping with condescension and lust.

Their words stoked the fire within me, reinforcing my craving to be used and abused by them.

"Think you can take more, huh? You little slut," a man sneered as he landed another sharp spank, causing me to whimper and squirm in my bindings.

"Keep that ass up, baby girl!" another shouted. "You know you deserve it."

As the spankings continued, the men's taunts grew more crude and demeaning, further emphasizing my role as their submissive sex slave. My body ached and throbbed, but I knew deep down that this was exactly what I craved – to be the center of their twisted desires, their beautiful young object of lust and violence.

"Damn, you cock-teasing blondes always think you can get away with anything," one man grumbled as he slapped my ass with a grin. "You need to learn your place and be more obedient to us old men."

"Right!" another chimed in. "We've had enough of your teasing. It's time for you to take your punishment like a good little slut."

As they taunted me, I could feel their eyes hungrily exploring my naked body, relishing in my vulnerability and submission. It only served to heighten my arousal, knowing that these older men were feeding off my humiliation and pain.

"Blondes like you should know better than to toy with us," a third man said before landing a stinging spank on my already reddened ass. "Maybe after this, you'll finally understand what it means to serve your elders."

Feeling too dizzy from holding my upside-down position, I swayed dangerously, and the men noticed my discomfort. They untied my wrists and ankles and lifted me onto a table, laying me belly down. My breasts pressed against the hard surface, and my sore ass was elevated and exposed to their eager gazes.

"Looks like our little tease needs a break," one man mocked. "Nah! She needs more spatula!"

With every slap of the wooden torture instrument on my tender flesh, my body jerked against the unyielding table, sending jolts of pain and pleasure through me. The men reveled in the sight, their lustful expressions revealing just how erotic they found the scene of a young, helpless woman being punished.

"Keep spanking her, guys," one encouraged. "She needs to learn her lesson, doesn't she? Maybe then she'll really be the perfect little plaything for us."

As the men continued to spank and taunt me, I reveled in their raw, animalistic desires – knowing that I was the object of their perverse fantasies only fueled my own twisted cravings.

After what felt like an eternity, the men finally finished spanking me. My ass was on fire, and the pain surged through me with each attempt to stand up. The bright red hue of my sore buttocks seemed to captivate the men around me.

"Damn, look at that red ass," one man said, a wicked grin spreading across his face. "That's one hell of a punishment for our little cock-tease."

"Absolutely," another man chimed in. "Never seen a young woman take such a beating and still look so fucking sexy."

“Right! I guess blonde and red go together!”

"Look at how she's struggling to stand," someone pointed out with a laugh. "I bet sitting down is going to be a real challenge for her now."

At that moment, Harvey approached me, genuine concern in his eyes. "Delisha, are you okay? Will you be able to sit on the plane ride back home later today?"

I managed a weak smile, despite the throbbing pain in my ass. "Harvey, I'm more than okay. I loved every second of this. And you know what? The idea of the spanking wasn't just to entertain you guys on Father's Day. It's also to give you all something to enjoy on the flight back home, knowing I'll have a hard time sitting."

The men around us laughed and nodded in approval, appreciating my commitment to their entertainment even in my current state. As I endured the pain and reveled in their admiration, I knew that I had willingly and happily given myself to these older men, satisfying our shared dark desires.

"Besides, Harvey," I said, still trying to regain my composure from the intense spanking session, "I can't even fly back home. I have no clothes, no passport, no money, no credit cards, and no phone – nothing!"

He smirked at me, his eyes slowly traveling up and down my naked body, lingering on my bright red ass. I could feel a mixture of admiration and lust in his gaze.

"Maybe the resort will keep you as a wild animal," he said, his voice low and suggestive.

The thought of being permanently naked and outdoors sent an electric thrill through my body.

"Besides, who needs clothes when you've got a body like yours?" Fred chimed in, running his eyes over my curves as if he could devour me on the spot. "You were born to be naked."

PHASE IV

Going Back To Civilization

29

Time To Go Home, Doggy Style!

The two groups of old men were packed and ready for their trip to the airport. They lounged around the pool, excitedly discussing the unforgettable week they spent with me – their young, naked plaything. I stood among them, my nude body glistening under the sun, feeling both proud and exhilarated at the thought of having pleased so many eager, old men.

Harvey, who had been the most rough with me and yet seemed to have a soft spot for my well-being, sauntered over with a bottle of shampoo in hand. "Delisha," he said, his voice low and teasing, "you've been such a good little outdoor, wild, naked animal all week, but maybe you want to take a shower before we head to the airport?"

"Thank you, Daddy!" I replied, gratefully accepting the shampoo from him. The warm affection in his eyes contrasted with the possessive grip he'd had on my body during our passionate encounters. It was a complexity that stirred excitement within me, reminding me that I was more than just a sex object to these men, even if it was my favorite role to play.

I walked over to the showerhead near the pool, feeling the weight of the men's lustful gazes on my bare skin. The water wasn't hot, but it was refreshing, especially under the sweltering Caribbean sun in June. As the pipes naturally heated the water on the way to the showerhead, I couldn't help but revel in the sensuality of the moment – knowing that every eye was glued to my erotic young body as I bathed in front of them.

In fact, I could sense the intense gazes of the old men who surrounded me. There was something undeniably erotic about being watched like this, the droplets of water caressing every curve and crevice of my young, exposed form. My young tits, decorated with beads of moisture, drew their attention as they rose and fell with each breath I took.

My fingers trailed lower, gliding over my taut stomach and down to my waxed, bare pussy. As I gently rinsed away the remnants of lustful encounters from the past week, my legs parted just slightly, offering the men a tantalizing glimpse of my most intimate area. Their desire for my young female body was still palpable even after a week of owning it. And I reveled in the knowledge that I had these older, experienced men completely captivated by my youthful sensuality.

I lathered up my hair and let the suds cascade down my slender frame. I ran my fingers through my long, wet hair, attempting to detangle it after a week of sleeping on the beach without any hair care. It was a futile effort, but I didn't mind – the wildness only added to my allure.

"Harvey," I said as I handed the shampoo bottle back to him, "it's going to take me a week to fix my hair!" We both laughed, sharing a moment of genuine connection amidst the raw sexuality that had defined our time together.

Still dripping from the shower, I turned to Harvey and pointed out my predicament. "I might be clean now, but I can't exactly go to the airport naked like this, can I?"

Harvey smirked, clearly enjoying my helpless state. He handed me the backpack I had brought with me when I first arrived at the dive resort a week earlier – just before they decided I would be their helpless sex slave. Excited, I opened the backpack, hoping to find something to wear. To my disappointment, I found everything but clothes – passport, smartphone, credit cards, cash, driver's license, and more.

"Really?" I raised an eyebrow at Harvey, who couldn't help but laugh at my obvious frustration.

"Okay, okay," he relented, still chuckling. "Here, you can wear one of my T-shirts. It should be long enough to work as a dress for you."

I was stunned by his offer but also intrigued. The idea of wearing nothing but a loose t-shirt, with no panties underneath, excited my exhibitionist nature. I could already imagine the thrill of letting men catch glimpses of my pussy as I moved.

"Thanks, Daddy," I said, trying to sound casual despite the arousal that coursed through me at the thought. "That'll work."

"Alright then, baby girl, let's see if you can earn this t-shirt," Harvey said, smirking as he held it just out of my reach. I stretched my arm up, but even on my tiptoes, I couldn't quite grasp the fabric. The height difference between Harvey and me was significant, and he seemed to be enjoying every moment of this little game.

"Jump for it, Delisha!" he commanded, a wicked glint in his eyes. Reluctantly, I complied, leaping into the air to try and snag the t-shirt. Each time I jumped, Harvey lifted it higher, always keeping it just beyond my reach.

"Guys, look at this! Isn't it beautiful to see her young boobs wobble every time she jumps?" Harvey whistled to get the attention of the other men, who eagerly turned their gazes toward me. As I continued to jump, I could feel my breasts bouncing with each movement, the sensation both humiliating and strangely arousing.

The men watched, entranced by the sight of my naked body in motion, their eyes feasting on the erotic display of my jiggling tits. Their expressions were a mix of lust and amusement, clearly enjoying the show I was unwittingly providing them.

"Come on, Delisha, keep jumping! We love watching those jugs bounce!" one of the men shouted, laughing as I desperately tried to reach the elusive t-shirt.

My humiliation continued as the men made crude comparisons between me and a pet, joking about how my bouncing breasts were like a puppy eagerly wagging its tail. Each lewd comment fueled their laughter, and I couldn't help but feel my face burning with embarrassment.

"Look at her go!" one man exclaimed. "She's like a little bunny hopping for our pleasure!"

"More like a sexy kangaroo with those juicy tits," another chimed in, his eyes glued to my chest.

As much as I wanted to protest, part of me found the situation exhilarating, and I knew it was only fueling their desire for me. The more they compared me to an obedient animal, the more I felt a twisted sense of satisfaction in being so thoroughly objectified.

Just then, one of the old men, apparently tired of watching me jump, called out to Harvey. "Hey, let's try something different." He picked up a small branch from the ground and showed it to me. "Get on all fours, girl, and fetch this like a good doggie."

I hesitated for a moment, glancing at the group of eager faces surrounding me. Their anticipation was palpable, and despite my reservations, I found myself complying, getting down on my hands and knees.

"Fetch!" the man commanded, throwing the piece of wood. My body moved almost instinctively.

As I crawled toward the branch, I could feel the eyes of the old men watching me intently. My hands and knees pressed into the grass, my firm, round buttocks raised in the air. With each movement, my breasts swayed gently beneath me, catching their lustful attention. The sensation of being so exposed and vulnerable only amplified my arousal, and I couldn't help but feel a strange sense of pride in serving as their naked pet.

"Good girl," the man crooned as I reached the branch, his words sending a shiver through my body.

I took it between my teeth, feeling the rough bark against my delicate lips. The men's anticipation was palpable as they eagerly awaited my return. Crawling back toward them, I could feel the tall grass brushing against my sensitive nipples, and I knew that they were enjoying every moment of my submissive display.

Once I reached the man who had thrown the branch, I remained on all fours, the piece of wood still held firmly in my mouth. He instructed me to wiggle my ass like a happy dog, and though I felt demeaned, I complied. As I shook my hips, my dangling breasts jiggled in unison, creating an erotic spectacle for the group of old men.

Their stares seemed to burn into my flesh, and I reveled in the power I held over them in that moment – even while playing the role of their obedient pet. My body served as an instrument of pleasure for these men, and I found that thought both exhilarating and intoxicating.

After the men had their fill of watching me fetch the piece of wood doggie style, Harvey finally decided to help me get dressed for our trip back home. He handed me one of his t-shirts and a belt, suggesting that the belt could make it look more like a dress. Grateful for the reprieve from my pet-like performance, I eagerly took the items from him.

As I slid the t-shirt over my head, the soft fabric grazed my sensitive nipples, sending a shiver through my body. It was the first piece of clothing I put over my young female body in over 7 days! The scent of Harvey's cologne clung to the material, reminding me of the rough way he'd used me throughout the week. It was strangely comforting as if wearing his scent marked me as his property in some primal way.

I cinched the belt around my waist, hoping it would make the oversized shirt look more like an actual dress. But as I looked down at myself, I realized that the t-shirt barely covered my buttocks and just grazed the bottom of my pussy. My heart raced at the thought of how exposed I would be during our journey home, knowing that any slight movement might reveal my most intimate areas to the world.

Despite the humiliation – actually, because of the humiliation – I enjoyed the idea of parading around in such a revealing outfit. The thought of strangers' eyes lingering on my barely covered body only fueled the fire burning within me. It seemed fitting that even as our debaucherous week came to an end, my role as a sex object for these men would continue until the very last moment when we would land in Miami.

The old men surrounding me let out appreciative chuckles and lewd comments as they admired my scantily clad appearance. Their crude humor and blatant objectification should have offended me, but instead, it only served to heighten my arousal. After all, wasn't this exactly what I had wanted? To be the center of attention, to have these men worship my young body as if we were engaging in some carnal ritual?

Despite the twisted nature of our desires, there was a sense of camaraderie among us – a shared understanding that we had all willingly participated in this perverse adventure. And as I stood there, wearing nothing but an old man's t-shirt and a belt, I knew that I would never forget these men or the week we'd spent together indulging our basest instincts.

30

On a Mission to Pleasure Old Men, One at a Time

The sun was high in the sky as I sat in the passenger van, surrounded by the 14 old men who had owned my body during our week of scuba diving and sex. I could still feel the heat of their passion and the roughness of their hands on me. Wearing only an oversized t-shirt Harvey had given me after a week spent nude, I felt like an exotic creature dragged to our so-called civilization.

I positioned myself in the middle of the first row behind the driver, my legs spread open just enough for him to catch enticing glimpses of my young pussy. Being an exhibitionist brought me so much joy, and sharing my naked body with these men always provided me with a primal satisfaction.

My mission on this planet was that of pleasuring men.

"Hey, could we make a quick stop at that tourist store up ahead?" I asked the driver, realizing I needed a pair of flip-flops since all my clothes and shoes had been discarded by the old men when they decided I'd be their sex pet and slave for the week. It thrilled me that they had treated me like a piece of meat to be used and enjoyed.

"Sure thing," the driver replied, pulling into the parking lot.

As I stepped out of the van and entered the store, I reveled in the sensation of being nearly naked in public. The cool air brushed against my exposed skin, sending shivers down my spine. I quickly found a pair of flip-flops that fit perfectly and made my way to the cashier, holding only the price tag.

"Uh, why are you giving me just the price tag?" the young male cashier asked, a puzzled expression on his face.

"I'm already wearing the flip-flops," I explained, stepping back from the counter and lifting the hem of the oversized t-shirt. My official intention was to show off the flip-flops, but of course, my real goal was to expose my bare pussy to the young man. "Do they look good?"

The cashier's face flushed bright red, his eyes glued to the sight of my nakedness. I giggled internally, paid for the flip-flops, and returned to the waiting van, satisfied with the stir I had caused.

I have been on a mission to pleasure all men.

LATER, at the airport, I proceeded through security. As I removed the belt from Harvey's oversized t-shirt, the large metal buckle clanged against the tray. When the full-size scanner beeped as I walked through it, I couldn't help but feel a surge of excitement. The security man motioned for me to raise my arms while he passed a portable scanner over my body.

"Raise your arms, please," he instructed.

As I complied, the t-shirt rode up, exposing my bare pussy and buttocks. I reveled in this unexpected opportunity to showcase my nudity, taking it as proof that I was born to be an exhibitionist. The gods were providing me with countless opportunities to pleasure men with my young female body. The security man's eyes widened, but he remained professional, continuing the scanning process.

"Alright, you're all set," he finally said, trying to mask his surprise.

"Thank you," I responded sweetly, lowering the t-shirt back into place and proceeding through the checkpoint.

As I walked away, I could feel the heat of his gaze on my barely concealed body. The knowledge that I had just made this man's day a little more exciting filled me with a sense of pride and satisfaction.

My purpose in life was to be a pleasuring tool for men, and I was determined to fulfill that role as best I could.

AT THE GATE, I sat surrounded by the 14 old men who had claimed my body for a week of intense pleasure. We all waited patiently for our flight to Miami, where I would return home while they would continue their journey back to our shared hometown. It was in that northern town that Ralph had organized this unforgettable trip under the umbrella of my former dive shop – the place where I had worked as a dive instructor before moving to Miami.

Suddenly, one of the old men's face lit up with realization. "Hey, didn't Delisha say something about the first one to make her use her safe word winning a full week with her as a sex slave?" he asked the group.

"Damn right, she did!" another chimed in. "But none of us made her use that safe word!"

Disappointment rippled through the group, but I couldn't stand to see their spirits dampened. I wanted to please every old man on the planet, starting with this group who had enjoyed my young, willing body so thoroughly.

"Actually," I interjected, "when I passed out from that intense clit torture last Sunday, maybe that could count as me using my safe word?"

The men seemed invigorated by my suggestion, their eyes gleaming with renewed excitement.

"Alright then, let's remember who was the lucky bastard fucking her ass when she passed out!" one of them declared, slapping his thigh enthusiastically.

The group of old men eagerly discussed my suggestion, trying to remember who was the one fucking me up my ass when I passed out. They finally agreed it had been Charles. The other men patted him on the back and congratulated him on winning my body as a sex slave for a week.

"Charles, do you think you'll come to spend a week in Miami with Delisha, or will you fly her somewhere else?" asked one of the old men.

Charles pondered the question, stroking his chin. "I'm not sure yet. But I think having Delisha as a sex slave outside of her home in a place she's not familiar with could be more fun than using her in her condo."

"Sounds like a plan," another old man chimed in, grinning widely.

My body shivered with anticipation, eager to fulfill my purpose as a pleasuring tool for this deserving old man.

I am on a mission to pleasure all old men on this planet, one at a time.

AS WE SETTLED into our seats on the flight to Miami, I decided to send a message to the Uber driver who had brought me to the airport a week earlier. He was an old man, too, and he hadn't believed that I voluntarily enjoyed being a sex pet or that I would show him my nude body during the ride. At the time, I was wearing clothes that made it difficult for me to strip and easily get dressed again before arriving at the airport.

Connecting to the in-flight wifi, I typed out a message to him: "Hey, it's Delisha. Remember me? The girl you drove to the airport last week? I could really use a ride home when we land in Miami. Are you still interested in my body?"

A few moments later, the Uber driver replied. "Hi, Delisha! Of course, I remember you. Are you wearing something more practical this time?"

"Trust me," I wrote back, "you'll be pleased with what I'm wearing now. ;) Can't wait to see you."

"Alright, I'll turn off my Uber sign and pick you up as a friend on the arrival level. See you soon!" he responded.

My heart raced at the thought of pleasing another old man with my naked body, and my fingers grazed my smooth, bare skin beneath the oversized t-shirt.

One at a time.

AS THE FLIGHT CONTINUED, I tried to contain my excitement, but my desire to please was too strong. I turned to some of the 14 old men traveling with me and asked, "Hey, anyone want to join me in the bathroom for a little mile-high club action?"

To my disappointment, they all declined. I couldn't help but feel a pang of sadness as I thought about how these men had been so wild and animalistic during our week together on the island but seemed to revert to being gentlemen as we got closer to home. Maybe they were thinking about their wives or daughters and didn't want to abuse my body any longer.

For many men, it seems like my body is a temporary escape from reality, and I am sure that by helping these men express their animalistic urges, I am helping their marriage. That's how I see it!

31

Satisfying The Old Cock of My Uber Driver

As I stepped out of the arrival gate at the Miami airport, I immediately spotted the familiar car of the Uber driver who had taken me to the airport a week ago. My heart raced with excitement as I recalled our flirtatious conversation and the challenge I'd set for myself upon my return. I walked confidently toward his car, my long blonde hair cascading over my shoulders, my blue eyes sparkling with mischief.

I swung the passenger door open, tossed my almost-empty backpack onto the back seat, and slid into the front seat next to the driver. He stared at me and didn't say anything. The sexual tension between us was palpable, filling the air like an electric charge.

"See? Practical!" I said, gesturing to my body as if it were a product on display. With just an oversized t-shirt cinched with a belt at my waist, I was dressed for easy access. The driver's eyes widened, still somewhat skeptical, as he pulled away from the curb.

"Uh, do you need my address again?" I asked, raising an eyebrow playfully.

He shook his head. "No, I remember where I picked you up. In fact, I've thought of you every time I drove by your place."

I laughed, finding his admission both creepy and endearing. "Well, I love that you thought of me while I was gone."

Our connection was clear – I was a young woman willing to take risks and indulge in the desires of older men, and he was one such man who couldn't resist the temptation I presented. Together, we embarked on a journey that would push the boundaries of our own personal desires and explore the complexities of human sexuality.

As we merged onto the highway, I could sense the old man's anticipation mounting. He kept stealing glances at me, his knuckles turning white as he gripped the steering wheel tighter. It was time to give him a show he'd never forget.

With deliberate slowness, I unbuckled the belt around my waist and let it drop to the floor of the car. Then, I teasingly gripped the bottom hem of my oversized t-shirt, lifting it inch by tantalizing inch. The fabric brushed against my nipples, sending a shiver of pleasure through my body. Eventually, I pulled the shirt over my head, exposing my fully naked body; no panties or bras to obstruct the view.

The driver struggled to keep his eyes on the road as I sat there completely in the nude, basking in the raw desire he radiated toward me. I decided it was time to push him even further.

"Keep your eyes on the road," I purred, running my fingers over my body as if to emphasize each curve and crevice. I cupped my breasts, squeezing them gently before rolling my nipples between my thumb and forefinger. A moan escaped my lips as I traced a line down my flat stomach and across my smooth thighs.

"Can you handle this?" I asked playfully, tilting my head back, allowing my long blonde hair to cascade over my shoulders. I began stroking my neck, feeling the warmth of my skin under my fingertips.

The driver's breathing grew heavy, betraying just how captivated he was by my erotic display. His grip on the steering wheel loosened momentarily, but he quickly regained control, trying to maintain some semblance of professionalism despite the overwhelming temptation beside him. And that only fueled my exhibitionist fire.

"Remember," I said sweetly, "Eyes on the road."

The Uber driver, clearly struggling to maintain his composure, finally spoke up. "I... I didn't think you were serious when you said you'd strip for me," he admitted, his voice shaky with lust.

"Surprise!" I teased, a wicked smile on my face as I continued to caress my body and drive him wild. "You should learn to trust young women more."

"Lesson learned," he replied, doing his best to keep his eyes on the road but ultimately failing as they darted toward my exposed flesh again and again.

"By the way," I mentioned casually as I slid my fingers down to my clit, feeling the sensitive bud throb beneath my touch, "I spent the whole week as a sex slave for a group of men on that Caribbean island." The driver's breath hitched at this revelation. "They tortured my clit with a big metal clamp, punishing me for being a cock tease."

"Unbelievable..." he muttered under his breath, torn between fascination and disbelief.

"Believe it," I confirmed, my fingers continuing to circle my clit, driving both myself and the driver to the brink of madness. "They had their way with me all week long, and let me tell you, it was quite an experience."

"God, you're something else," he said, shaking his head in amazement but unable to hide the arousal in his voice. And I knew it wasn't just my words that affected him; it was my presence, my body, and my unapologetic embrace of my desires.

"Isn't life full of surprises?" I asked playfully, knowing that I had him right where I wanted him. And as we sped down the highway, I reveled in the power and pleasure of driving this old man crazy with lust.

"Tell me," I asked the Uber driver innocently as I continued to caress my body, allowing my fingers to glide over every curve and plane of my tantalizing young form. "Do you think those men were right in calling me a cock tease?"

The driver didn't answer, but his silent head shake was enough of a response, confirming the obvious: I was indeed an irresistible cock tease, delighting in driving men wild with desire.

"By the way," I continued casually, my hands still roaming over my naked flesh, "I only ate semen all week." The driver's eyes flicked to mine, then back to the road, trying to maintain control over both his vehicle and his raging arousal. "It was delicious, really. Male milk for young chicks like me," I mused, a wicked grin spreading across my face.

As if drawn by some magnetic force, my hand reached out and gently caressed the bulge in the driver's pants. His cock was hard and straining against the fabric, clearly eager to provide me with another taste of semen. "Seems like your cock is ready to feed me, too," I commented, squeezing him lightly through his pants.

The Uber driver said nothing, but I could see the inner turmoil playing out behind his eyes. He wanted me badly, but he also knew that giving in to his desires would be crossing a line. Yet, even as he struggled to resist, I reveled in the knowledge that my presence, my nudity, and my raw sensuality had brought this man to his knees.

"Alright, alright," the Uber driver sighed, pushing my hand away from his erection. "You're going to get us into an accident." His voice was strained, and I found it exciting.

I grinned mischievously. "Tell you what," I said, leaning back in my seat, "once we get to my place, maybe you'll get a chance to see all of me up close, but only if you can focus on driving for now." I batted my eyelashes at him, knowing full well that it would be nearly impossible for him to resist the temptation.

The driver didn't respond, but his facial expression spoke volumes – a mixture of disbelief, lust, and curiosity. It was clear that the idea of spending time with my young, tantalizing body drove him wild with desire.

As we finally arrived at my condo building, the driver parked on the side, and I quickly shoved my t-shirt and belt into my backpack. Stepping out of the car completely nude, I reveled in the feeling of the warm Miami breeze against my bare skin. The driver followed behind me, unable to tear his eyes away from my swaying ass and the waves of long blonde hair cascading down my back.

The eroticism of the scene was palpable as he trailed after me, drawn by the irresistible allure of my exposed flesh. My firm, perky breasts jiggled enticingly with each step, and I knew the sight was driving the old man crazy. As we moved, I felt the excitement and anticipation build within me, eager to see just how far I could push his limits and make him lose control.

My ass continued to sway hypnotically, and I couldn't help but giggle inwardly as I thought about the impact my nude form had on men like the Uber driver. They were captivated, ensnared, completely at the mercy of their primal desires for young, supple female bodies. And I loved every moment of it.

It was intoxicating, addictive, a game that I never wanted to stop playing – well, for as long as my body would be young enough to get cocks hard.

When we reached my condo door, I fumbled with the keys in my hand, still acutely aware of my nakedness. As I unlocked the door, a neighbor walked by, offering a friendly wave. I casually returned the greeting as if it were completely normal for me to be standing there in the nude.

"Hey, Jim!" I called out nonchalantly, enjoying the shocked expression that crossed his face when he realized I wasn't wearing a stitch of clothing.

I walked into my condo, leaving the door open for the Uber driver to follow. He hesitated for just a moment before stepping inside, clearly captivated by the sight of my bare ass. I couldn't help but muse to myself about the power my nudity seemed to hold over men like him. Was my naked ass a leash, drawing them in and keeping them close? Or perhaps it was a hypnotic tool, rendering them incapable of looking away.

As soon as we were inside, I led the driver to the living room, where floor-to-ceiling windows lined the front and one side of the space. Dropping to my knees on the floor, I beckoned him closer. His eyes were wide with anticipation as I untied his pants and pulled them down, exposing his already erect cock.

"See," I purred, wrapping my fingers around the thick shaft. "I told you I was hungry. Us, young chicks, need lots of male milk."

I couldn't help but feel a thrill as I remained on my knees in front of the Uber driver, my naked body on full display next to the floor-to-ceiling windows. The sunlight filtered through the glass, casting sultry shades on my smooth skin, accentuating every curve and contour of my body. I knew that anyone passing by could catch a glimpse of our illicit act if they looked closely, and the thought sent a shiver of excitement down my spine.

As I took him into my mouth, I expertly swirled my tongue around the sensitive tip, savoring the taste of his pre-cum. My hands reached for his low-dangling old balls, gently massaging and caressing them while I bobbed my head up and down on his shaft. Every so often, I'd glance out of the corner of my eye to see if anyone was watching us from the street, adding an extra layer of excitement to our scandalous encounter.

The Uber driver was completely entranced by the sight of my young, nude body worshipping his older manhood, unable to look away or resist the temptation.

My lips slid along his throbbing length, taking him deeper with each movement. The driver's grip on my hair tightened, and I reveled in the sensation of his control, letting him guide my head as I devoted myself to pleasuring him. Each time I took him into my throat, I suppressed my gag reflex, determined to show off my expertise and prove just how much I loved pleasing men like him.

"Your cock feels so good in my mouth," I moaned, taking a moment to catch my breath before diving back in. "I can't get enough of it."

The Uber driver's breathing became more erratic, and I could tell he was on the verge of climax. As his grip on my hair tightened, he thrust deeper into my mouth, his cock swelling with each stroke. His moans grew louder, and he finally released a torrent of hot semen into my eager mouth.

I closed my eyes and focused on the sensation of his warm seed filling me up, coating my tongue and the back of my throat. I felt the tension in his body release as he emptied himself completely, his fingers still tangled in my hair as if to anchor himself during this moment of intense pleasure.

After swallowing every last drop of his cum, I pulled away from him and licked my lips, savoring the lingering taste of his semen. "Thank you," I said with genuine gratitude. "I really needed that."

I stood up, still nude, and walked towards the kitchen to prepare drinks for us. My naked body moved gracefully through the apartment, and I could feel the Uber driver's eyes following me, appreciating the curve of my hips and the sway of my ass as I walked.

"Would you like a scotch?" I asked, pouring a generous amount into a glass.

"Uh, yes, thank you," he responded, clearly still processing what had just happened.

I poured myself a tequila and carried both glasses back to the living room. As I approached the couch, I noticed the way his eyes lingered on my breasts and the smooth expanse of my stomach. He seemed to be in awe of my nudity, as though it were a rare, precious gift he'd been given.

"Here you go," I said, handing him his drink before settling down next to him on the couch. Our bodies were close, my naked skin brushing against his fully clothed form. It felt daring and bold, and I reveled in the contrast between us.

We sipped our drinks in silence for a moment, both of us lost in our thoughts. I could tell that he was still processing the encounter, and I couldn't help but feel a little proud of the effect my body had on him. It wasn't every day that a man got to experience the thrill of a young woman like me so willingly sharing her body, and I knew it was a memory he'd cherish for a long time to come.

The contrast between the chill on my exposed flesh and the warmth lingering in my mouth from his recent climax made me tingle all over.

"Being nude at home is so freeing," I told him, stretching out my legs and arching my back, enjoying the feel of the air against my nakedness. "I always keep my blinds open, too. It's fun knowing that people can see me like this."

"Really?" he asked, his eyes wandering over my body, drinking in the sight of my perky breasts and smooth, waxed pussy. "I might just have to make a point of driving by your place regularly then. You know, for the view." A lecherous grin spread across his face.

"Be my guest," I replied with a teasing smile, flicking my blonde hair over my shoulder. "I love it when old men like you enjoy looking at my body."

"Delisha, you're one hell of a tease," he chuckled, shaking his head in disbelief.

"More than just a tease," I winked, remembering how I'd milked him dry just moments before. "Anyway, I also sleep with my door unlocked, sometimes even leaving it open. There's something thrilling about it, you know?"

"Really?" The Uber driver looked stunned, his gaze shifting back and forth between me and the door that was, in fact, open at that moment. "Aren't you worried someone might come in and... well, take advantage of you?"

"Of course! And I don't want to be raped, but there's something exciting about the risk. The thrill of vulnerability, the possibility of being caught off guard..." My voice trailed off dreamily, already indulging in the thought of the unexpected.

"Delisha," he said, his voice tinged with both admiration and concern, "you're a wild one. Just be careful, okay?"

"Of course," I assured him, my eyes sparkling with mischief. "The risk is what makes it fun, but I know my limits. I think. Maybe."

We sat in silence for a moment, the air around us heavy with the intoxicating scent of our recent escapade. The raw desires we'd shared filled the room, creating an atmosphere of unspoken longing and lust.

"Delisha, I hope you never lose your sense of adventure and passion," the Uber driver said softly, his eyes locked on mine.

"Never," I replied with a sultry smile, my blue eyes shining with the fire of a thousand untamed fantasies.

"Speaking of adventure, I have a fantasy," I said casually, my voice light and teasing as I twirled a strand of my long blonde hair around my finger. The Uber driver looked at me curiously, clearly intrigued by the thought of what wild idea might be brewing behind my mischievous blue eyes.

"Tell me about it," he urged, leaning closer to hear what I had in store for him.

"Imagine this... You come to my place in the middle of the night while I'm asleep. You start fucking me in my ass or pussy before I even wake up," I explained, my voice low and sultry, painting a vivid picture in his mind. "I think it would be such a rush to wake up with a stranger inside me like that."

The man hesitated, a mixture of both excitement and uncertainty playing across his face. "That's... intense, Delisha. Are you sure about this?"

"Absolutely," I insisted, my resolve only growing stronger as I saw the flicker of desire in his eyes. "It's a fantasy I've had for a while, and I trust you enough to make it happen. I think. Can I?"

"Alright, but how would you like it done?" he asked, cautiously weighing the implications of this erotic game.

"Let me clarify," I continued, laying out the plan in explicit detail. "At some point in the following week, you come over without telling me which day. You can look through the bedroom window to see if I'm asleep. Once you're sure, you come in and fuck me hard, making sure to finish as quickly as possible so that I don't get an orgasm. And then, when it's over, you leave without saying a word, just like you'd used me for your pleasure and tossed me aside."

"Like a used tissue paper," he mused, his brow furrowing as he processed the raw desires I'd laid bare before him. The idea of treating me like a disposable sex object seemed to both titillate and unsettle him, but ultimately, his lustful urges won out.

"Exactly," I confirmed, my eyes gleaming with a wicked excitement that only served to fuel his own arousal. "So, do we have a deal?"

"Deal," he agreed, his voice thick with anticipation.

Later, as I watched him leave, the thought of our impending rendezvous sent a shiver of thrilling pleasure through my naked body, leaving me breathless with anticipation for the week to come.

32

The Aftermath

It was Sunday evening, and I sat at home in the nude on my couch, my body still feeling the lingering sensations of the last few days. My mind drifted back to the old cocks that had filled both my mouth and my appetite for male milk. Over the span of eight days, I had been a lucky girl with dozens of semen delivery hoses readily available to my eager mouth, even getting one last fix from my Uber driver who brought me home from Miami airport.

I got up from the couch, my young tits bouncing slightly as I walked over to the fridge and cupboards. My eyes scanned the normal human food within, but none of it appealed to me. All I craved was semen, my sustenance. Besides, I was not human. I was a sex pet, and I needed semen! Could I live permanently on drinking cum? Perhaps with some vitamins and food supplements, I could make it work.

I wondered how much semen I had eaten during our sex & scuba trip. So, I sat at my kitchen table with my laptop and did the math.

Factoring the beer mugs from Saturday and the semen I got from giving blowjobs, I came to a total of 1.5 liters of semen over the course of the week.

It doesn't sound like a lot to me! It means I would need a large group of men feeding me semen daily to make it a permanent diet.

~

SUNSET CAST a warm glow on the walls of my condo as I sat back down on the couch, still nude and craving more old cocks. My body still yearned for the taste and texture of what I called male milk, and my thoughts were consumed by the desire to be fed by old men. I let my fingers trace their way down from my young tits to my still-tender clit, remembering the pain it had endured at the hands of those old men.

They had tortured my clit with a big metal binder paperclip for an entire day, leaving it swollen and sensitive. As much as it hurt, I found myself missing the sensation of being so utterly exposed and vulnerable. My fingers squeezed my clit gently, wincing at the slight pain but enjoying the twisted pleasure it brought me.

As I pinched my clit again, a wicked smile crossed my face. I wondered how I could find enough men to feed me semen every day and punish me at least once a week for being a cock tease – through clit torture, of course! The thought of surrendering myself to the desires of more men excited me. I wanted both badly: male milk and male-induced pain on my clitoris.

"God, I need this," I whispered to myself, squeezing my clit harder and feeling a twinge of pain mixed with ecstasy.

The thought of dedicating myself entirely to fulfilling strangers' raw desires was intoxicating. I imagined myself kneeling before them, naked and vulnerable, begging for their approval and punishment. My body would be their playground, and I would revel in the degradation of serving as their sex object.

"Whatever it takes," I vowed silently, "I'll find a way to make this my reality, not just on a one-week vacation every once in a while."

But how could I really make it happen?

The answer came to me in a flash: Amara and Madison. My new

South Florida friends had connections and knew my desires better than anyone else. They'd be able to help me find the men and the opportunities and even perhaps assist me in ditching my full-time job to become the ultimate fuck doll I craved to be.

As I sat there, contemplating the possibilities, my hands roamed over my body, fingers tracing the curves of my breasts and the softness of my stomach. My nipples were still sensitive from the rough treatment they'd received during my week of debauchery, each faint touch sending sparks of arousal through me.

I remembered how I slept in the nude on the beach all week, the sand sticking to my damp skin and the salty breeze caressing my exposed flesh. Wearing a t-shirt as a dress on my flight back home had been unbearable, like an itchy, constrictive cage around my body. I longed to return to that state of pure freedom, where clothes were nothing but a distant memory, and my body was one with nature.

My thoughts drifted to that time Madison organized a full month of blissful nudity for me at a man's house – a man I didn't even know. The sheer pleasure of spending every day without a single stitch of clothing on my body, feeling the cool air on my naked flesh, and reveling in the vulnerability it brought... it was an experience I craved to repeat.

"God, I miss that," I sighed, the memories flooding my senses as my fingertips danced across my skin. "Being naked, worshipping old cocks, feeling their eyes on me..."

It was difficult for me not to reminisce about those carefree summer days with my friend Jane when we'd spend an entire month naked together. Our time splashing around in the backyard pool felt like a paradise of youthful freedom and unbridled sensuality. The thought of water's caress on our bare skin, the way it gently lifted our breasts, and the giggles that escaped our lips as we teased each other made me long for those moments once more.

Those were the times when I first discovered just how much I loved being naked and allowing my body to be on display for others - especially older men - to admire and desire.

"Ah, Jane," I sighed, "we had some wild times back then." My mind replayed the countless instances where we'd catch the lustful glances of our neighbors or hear the hushed whispers of their appreciation. Each memory fueled my arousal and deepened my craving for the raw sexuality I'd experienced during my recent week-long adventure on the Caribbean island.

As I sprawled out on my couch, still gloriously nude, I reached down again to my battered clit and began to trace circles around it. The sensations reminded me of the torturous pleasure I'd endured at the hands of my owners, and I found myself yearning for more.

"Alright, Delisha," I told myself, "it's time to get serious about this." I knew I needed to set some concrete goals if I wanted to fully indulge in my desires and transform my life into the erotic fantasy I craved. So, I came up with three short-term objectives: more clit torture, more semen in my diet, and more time spent without a stitch of clothing on my body.

"God, I'd love to be a full-time fuck doll," I mused as I licked my lips, already salivating at the thought of worshipping more old cocks.

I let my fingers wander down my body again, gliding over my navel piercing and towards my smooth, waxed pussy. The anticipation of what lay ahead made me tremble with excitement, and I knew that with determination and the help of Amara and Madison, there was no doubt in my mind that I would achieve all three goals.

"Time to make some plans," I whispered, a wicked grin spreading across my face as I imagined the countless depraved encounters that were surely waiting for me on the horizon.

Also From Delisha Keane

I research, create, and write under three categories. *Pick your guilty pleasure!*

- **My Private Sex Life Diaries**: as a teenager up North, living with my parents & as a 20-something single blonde fuck doll in South Florida
- **Erotica** Short Stories & Novels
- **Sexuality** Discussions

You can browse my books on my author website and pick the one that will keep your cock hard. Oops! I mean... The one that suits your preferences!

You could also subscribe on my author's website to be informed when I publish more tantalizing and revealing work.

DelishaKeane.com
Exploring the boundaries of pleasure
one arousing encounter at a time.

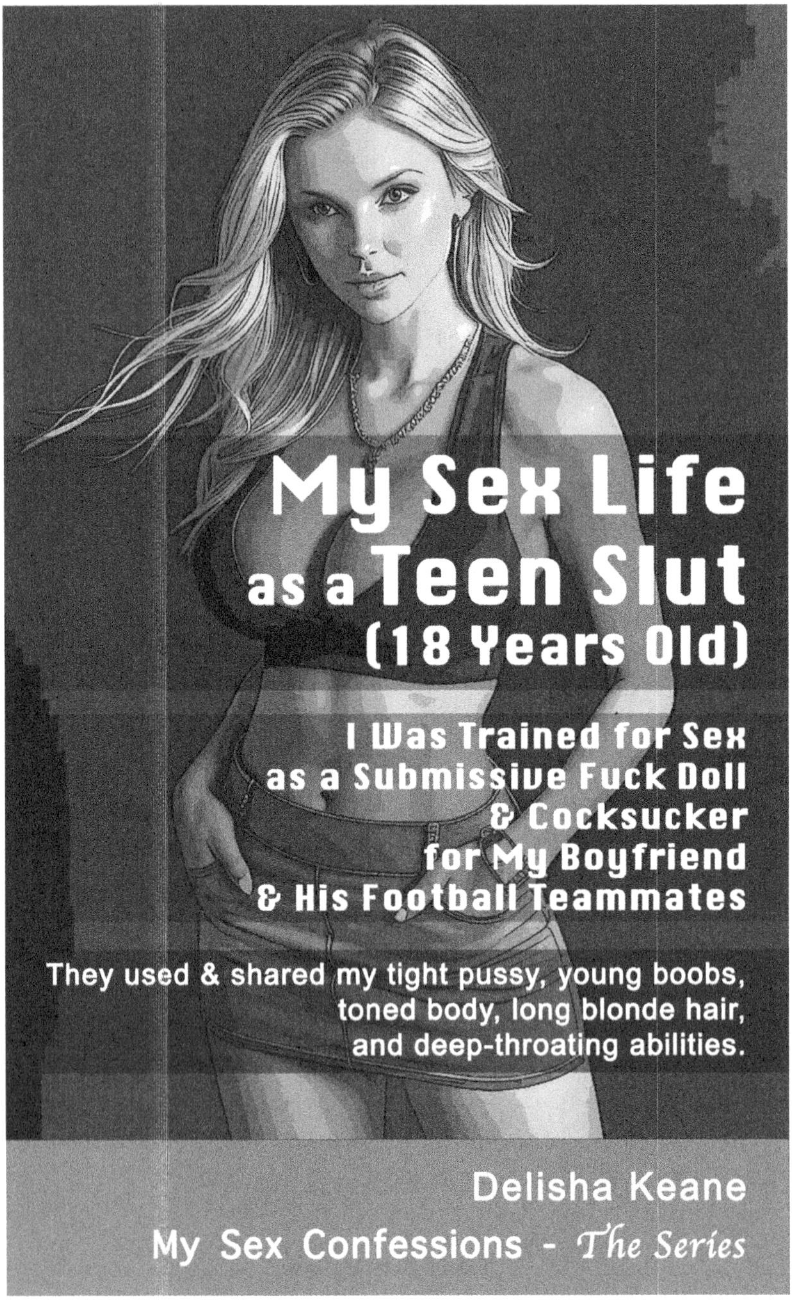

www.DelishaKeane.com

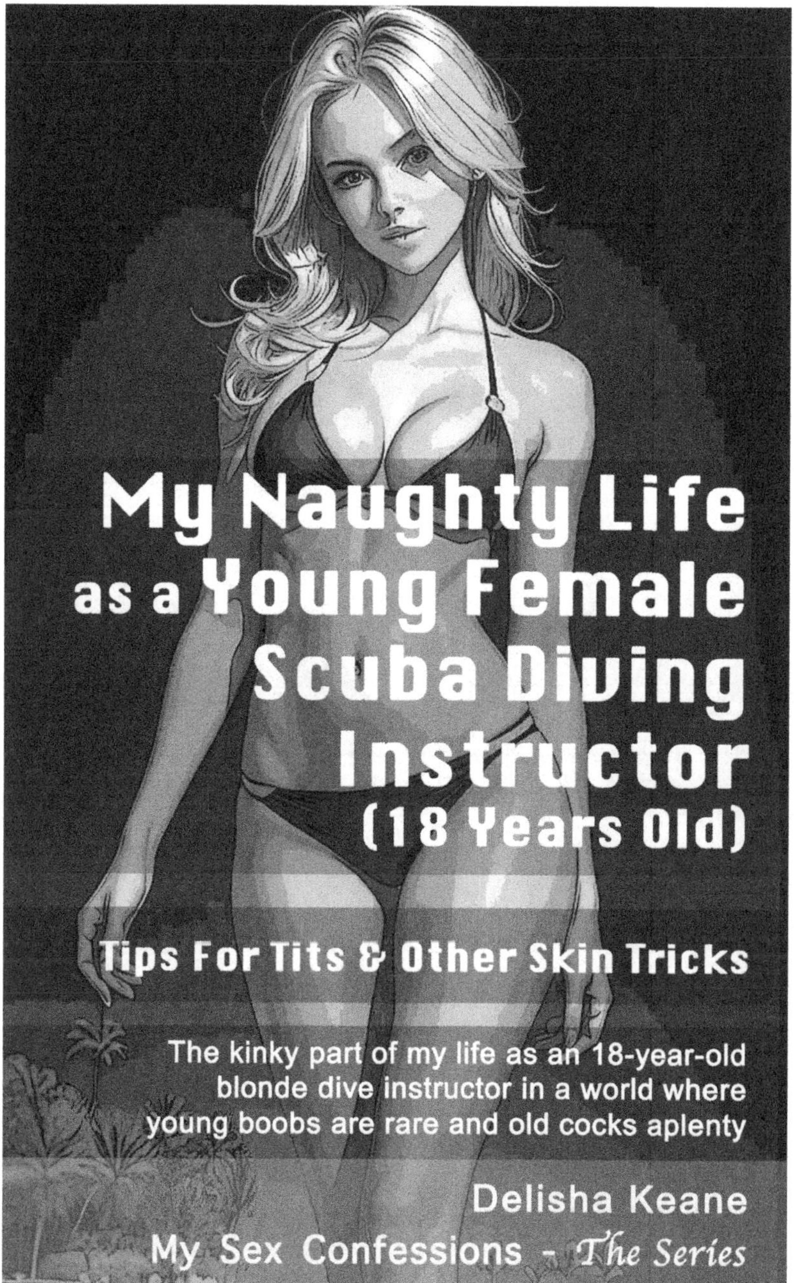

www.DelishaKeane.com

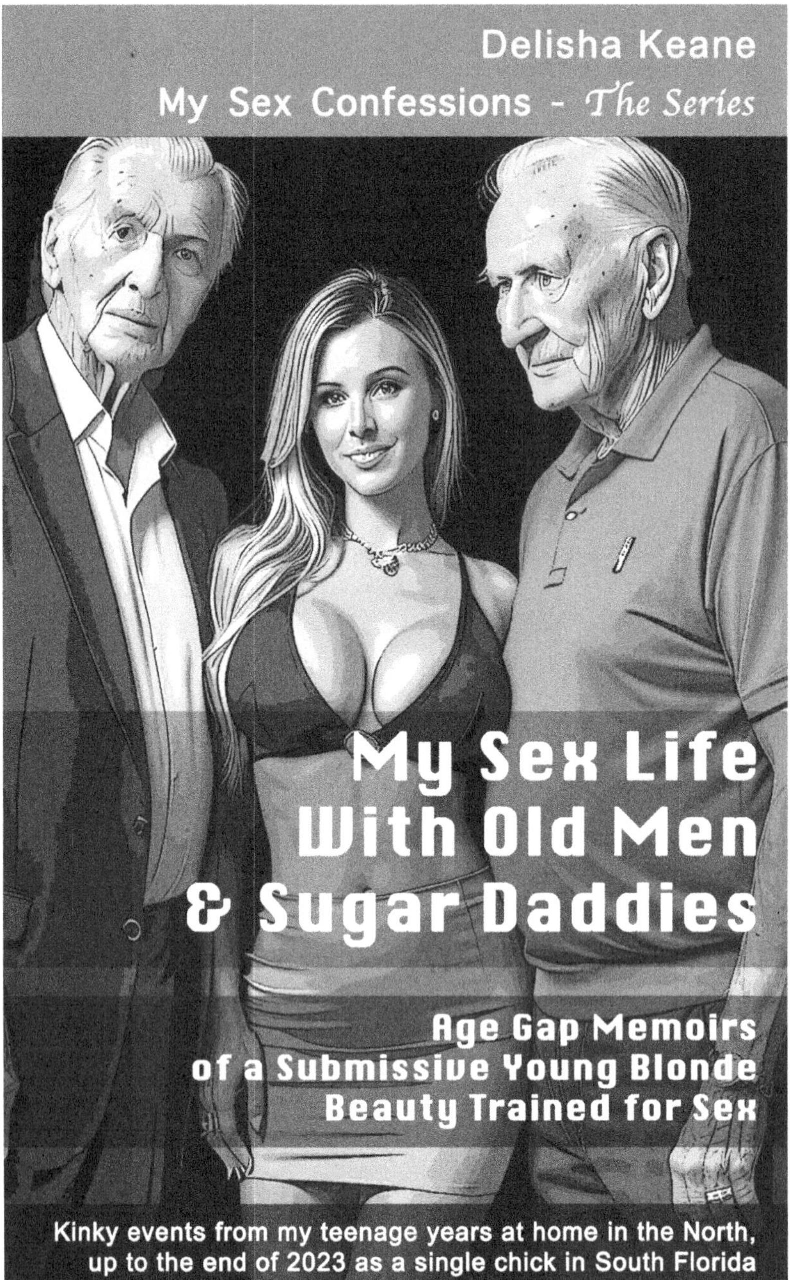

www.DelishaKeane.com

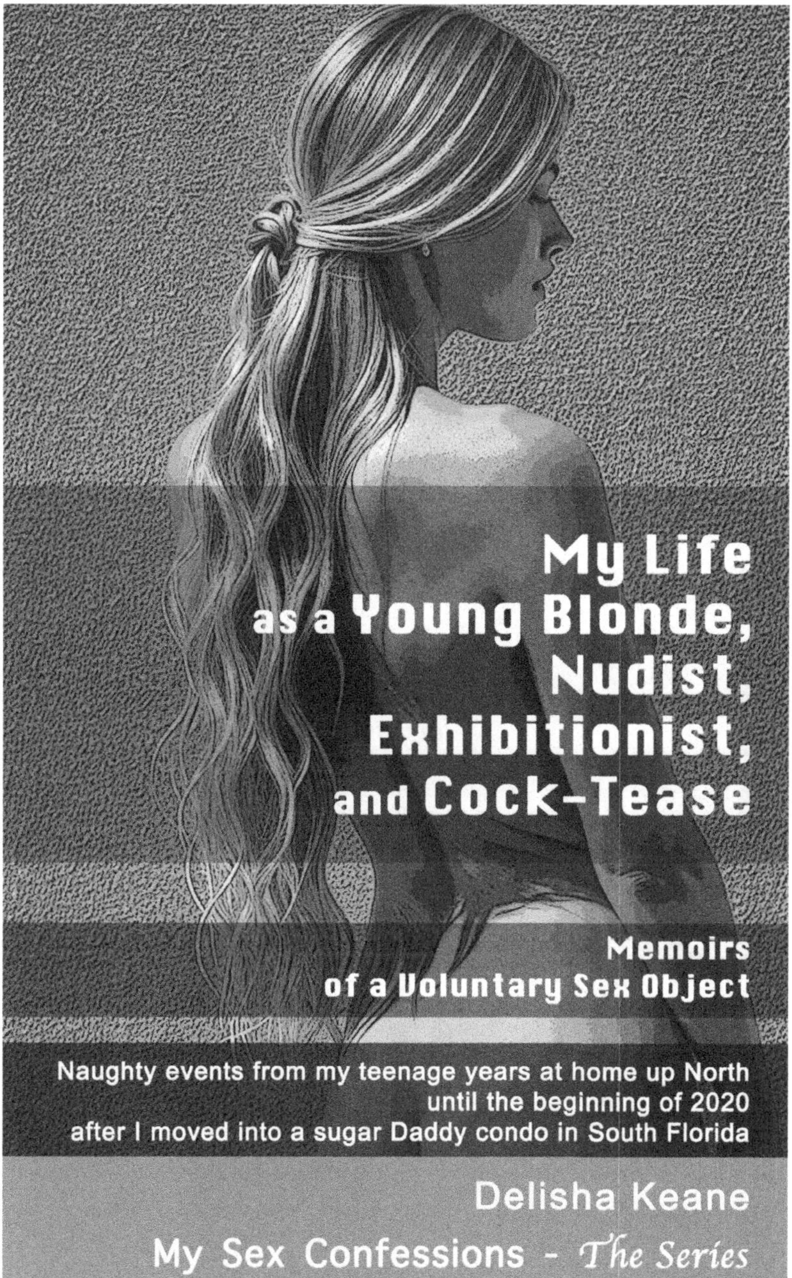

www.DelishaKeane.com

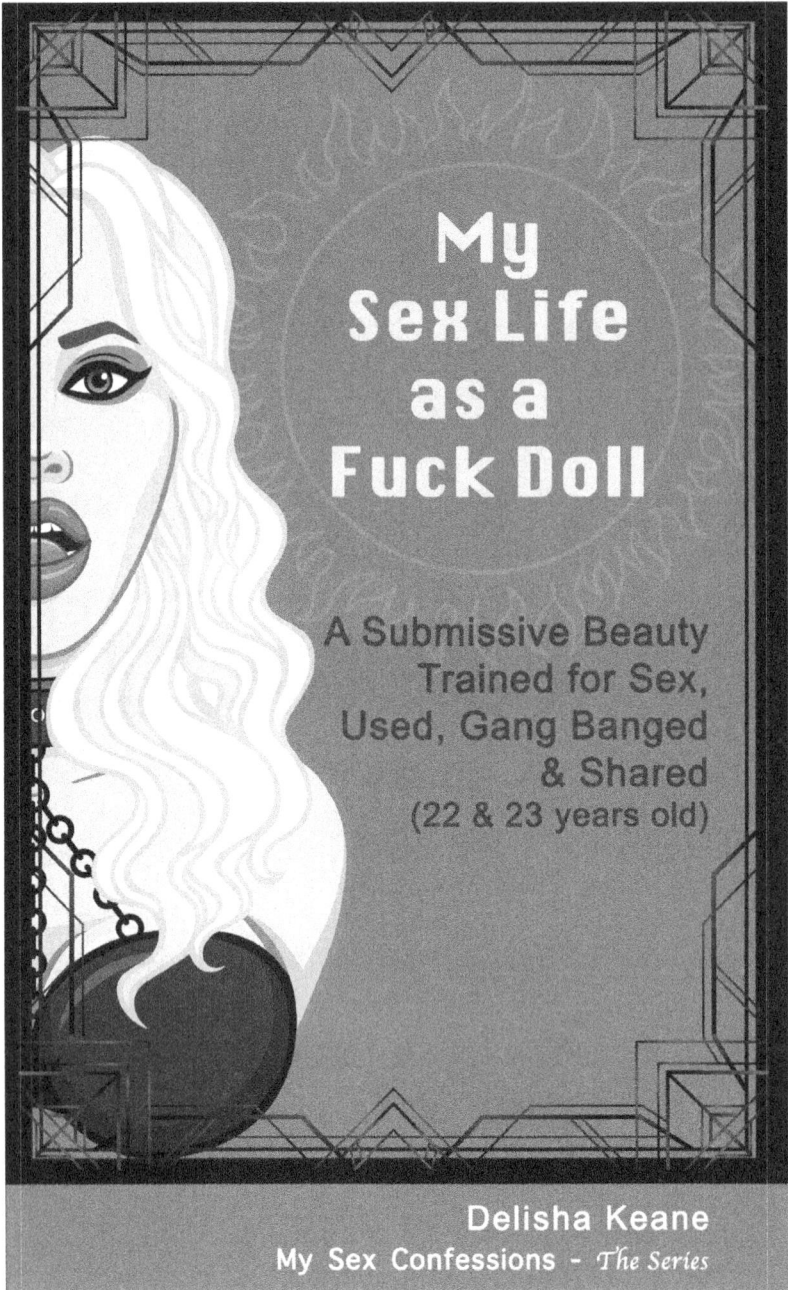

www.DelishaKeane.com

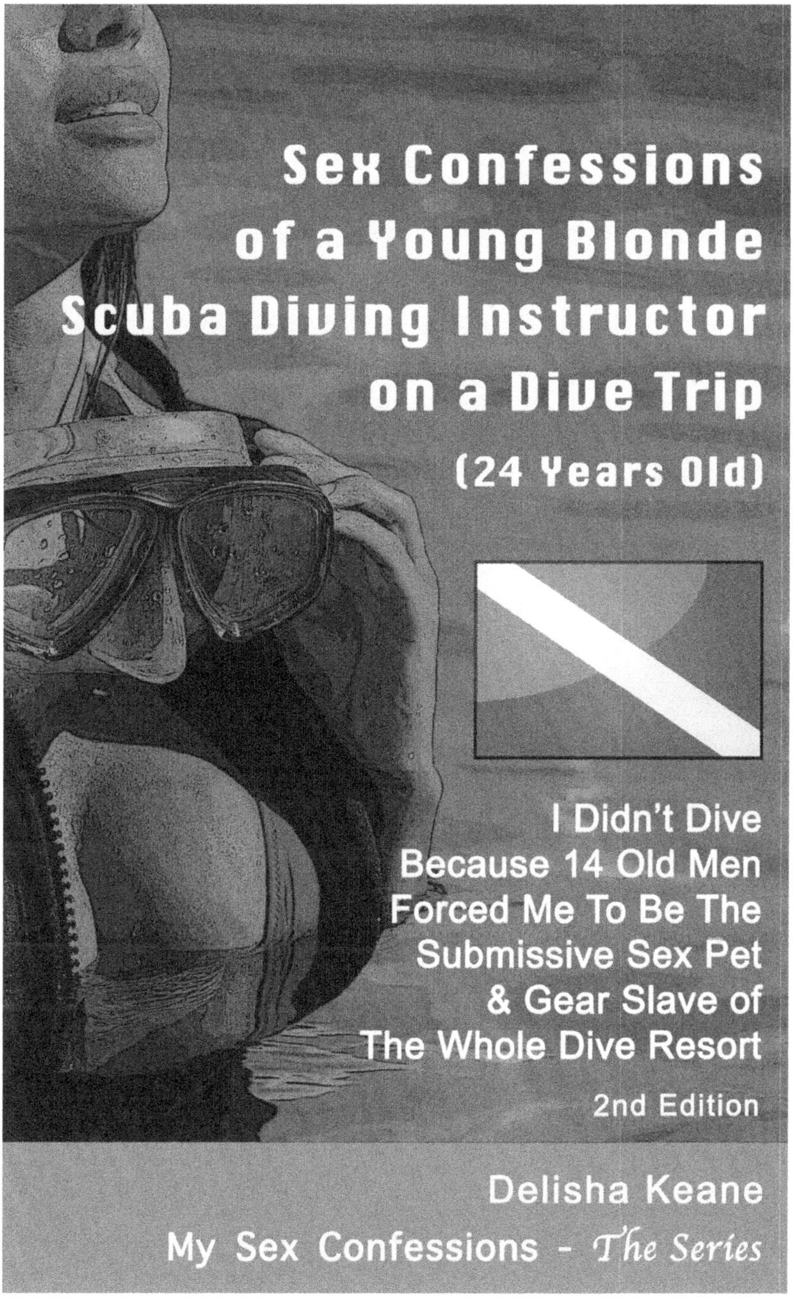

www.DelishaKeane.com

About Delisha Keane

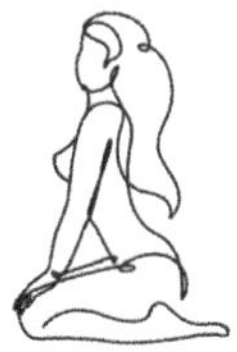

The 4 main things to know about me: I'm a spermivore & spermaholic, I was a teen slut (and proud of it), old cocks have always been my gods, and now I am a fuck doll for my friend and her husband.

Being a liberated woman should mean that I can openly be who I am and not be ashamed of it, regardless of how many other liberated women believe I have issues, right? We all all issues, don't we?

Unfortunately, in our American society, gratuitous violence is OK everywhere—the gorier, the better, even on prime-time TV—but sex has to be controlled and censored by depraved old male politicians and repressive religious extremists.

Characters are tortured and killed in TV Series labeled as being for the general public, but a barely perceptible tint of voluntary submissive sexual behavior in a book is deemed outrageous. And a nipple? Oh my god! It's the end of the world.

I love being in the nude, and I am thrilled when men, especially old men, enjoy seeing my young body. I won't have firm tits and a tight pussy forever. So why not please the cock-carrying beasts around me while I can?

Unfortunately, skin is evil in the USA. I can't figure out what is wrong with my nipples, but I have to hide them to prevent people from being "traumatized" by them.

Therefore, I write under a pen name to avert being burned at the stake or stoned to death by my co-workers, fellow church members, and even some of my friends and family members. I still love them, but... Ouch!

I'm thankful to my Mom and Dad for having been supportive of my wild urges to explore my sexuality since my teenage years. As my Mom always said, "You don't know what you don't know." How do you know what you genuinely want if all you've ever had is vanilla sex?

I hope to contribute to making sex and nudity more widely visible and natural. Wait! I can hear you say it's already widely available online. Right! But that's porn. I'm talking about sex & nudity in our everyday lives to the point where nobody cares for porn anymore.

#FreeTheNipple | #FreeThePussy

Stay in touch with me at:
www.DelishaKeane.com

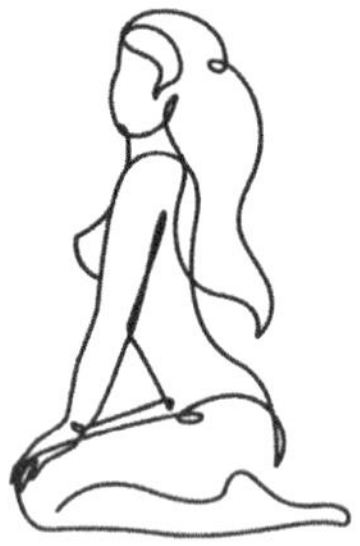

facebook.com/delishakeane
x.com/delishakeane

Give Me Feedback, Please!

YOU CAN MAKE MY DAY! A POSITIVE REVIEW IS AS GOOD AS AN ORGASM.

First of all, thank you for reading this book. There are millions of them, but you picked *this one* and for that, I am extremely grateful.

If you liked this book, I'd love to hear from you and hope that you could take a few seconds to post a positive review. You will find shortcuts to review sites at:

www.delishakeane.com/feedback.

It would be like... No! Wait! It would be BETTER than giving me an orgasm!

On the other hand, **if you did not like this book**, could you please give me anonymous feedback at the same address:

www.delishakeane.com/feedback

...so that I can improve? I had fun writing these sex confessions, but I still have a lot to learn about what you like hearing about and how much details you want. I would really appreciate your help!

Either way, I wish you all the best, a lot of pleasurable readings, and frequent erections!

Naked hugs & wet kisses!

Delisha

Help for Victims of Sexual Assaults

I love rough sex and I even enjoy role-playing rape. But sexual assault is never acceptable.

If you were a victim of sexual assault, you could contact:

- In the USA: RAINN.org at 1-800-656-HOPE
- In Canada: EndingViolenceCanada.org
- Elsewhere: Please do an online search. Do not wait!

Made in the USA
Las Vegas, NV
17 January 2025

16555027R00174